HOW TO
SUCCEED
NEW GRADUATE NURSING
JOB INTERVIEW
& BACHELOR OF NURSING
CLINICAL PLACEMENT?

MOHAN SANGRAULA

(Registered Nurse, NSLHD, Sydney, Australia)

BALBOA.
PRESS

A DIVISION OF HAY HOUSE

Balboa Press books may be ordered through booksellers or by contacting:

Balboa Press
A Division of Hay House
1663 Liberty Drive
Bloomington, IN 47403
www.balboapress.com.au
1 (877) 407-4847

Because of the dynamic nature of the Internet, any web addresses or links contained in this book may have changed since publication and may no longer be valid. The views expressed in this work are solely those of the author and do not necessarily reflect the views of the publisher, and the publisher hereby disclaims any responsibility for them.

The author of this book does not dispense medical advice or prescribe the use of any technique as a form of treatment for physical, emotional, or medical problems without the advice of a physician, either directly or indirectly. The intent of the author is only to offer information of a general nature to help you in your quest for emotional and spiritual well-being. In the event you use any of the information in this book for yourself, which is your constitutional right, the author and the publisher assume no responsibility for your actions.

Any people depicted in stock imagery provided by Thinkstock are models, and such images are being used for illustrative purposes only. Certain stock imagery © Thinkstock.

Print information available on the last page.

ISBN: 978-1-5043-0560-0 (sc)
ISBN: 978-1-5043-0561-7 (e)

Balboa Press rev. date: 02/08/2017

"Inside the book, you will find life- changing inspiration and successful secrets for bachelor of nursing students who aspire to succeed in new graduate nursing job interviews and clinical placement to become a registered nurse in Australia including an effective interview preparation technique and some important questions and answers example demonstrations".

A Lotus flower begins the journey at the bottom of the muddy pond, then slowly emerges towards the surface, bursting out of the water into a beautiful blossom. As like lotus, we as a student despite the challenges, equipped with knowledge, wisdom, experiences and skill and by overcoming the adversity need to move towards success, happiness and containment for self and others. If you practice the ideas mentioned in the book in a daily basis, your life will blossom as like Lotus flower.

"Be like A Lotus Flower Who Even Thrives In Challenge And Adversity"

PREFACE

The purpose in writing this book is to identify possible pitfalls in the professional experience placement and determine possible solutions to make the student's journey successful. The experiences I encountered were evidence-based. It also gives you some insights and provides some techniques to successfully secure a new graduate nursing program in Australia or outside. From my bottom of the heart, I would like to thank the university, lecturer, facilitator and preceptors who were directly or indirectly involved in enhancing my learning and making me successful in completing the professional experience placement (PEP) and securing the New Graduate Nursing program successfully. I have utilized the various resources to complete the book, and I have acknowledged them through references as much as possible. I would also like to acknowledge Smeltzer and Bare's *Textbook of Medical Surgical Nursing* which helped me to link bachelor of nursing theory to practice. I wish good luck to all the students for their future endeavours. Thank **You.**

ABOUT SUCCESS

Alexander Graham Bell, the inventor of the telephone, said, "Concentrate all your thoughts upon the work at hand. The sun's rays do not burn until brought to a focus." It means that success can be achieved if you focus on one single thing. He further stated that there is such power he cannot tell exactly what is it but he knows that it exists and it becomes available only when you are in that state of mind in which you know exactly what you want and are fully determined not to quit until you get it.

To succeed in any field and for everyone I would like to share the most suitable definition I have ever read which is in the book *Think Like a Winner* written by Dr Walter Doyle Staples. He has a quote from an interview with a Texas oil billionaire. He mentioned in his book H. L "Bunker" Hunt, the Texas oil billionaire, rose from being a bankrupt cotton farmer at age 32 during the Depression to earning more than one billion dollars per year by age 56. When asked in an interview about the secret of his success, Hunt replied that he believed there were only two things necessary to succeed. The first was that you need to decide exactly what is it you want. This is the starting point and, in his estimation, this is where most people fail. They never decide what is it they want. He observed that most people wander through life wanting a great many things but not wanting any one thing more than all the rest. They end up settling for far less than what could be theirs. Once you decide what you want, he continued the second thing you must do is determine the price you have to pay to get it, then resolve to pay that price. But many who get past the first step never get to the second. They never realize there is a price you need to pay for success" (Staples 1991, p 174). Therefore, it is your responsibility to decide what is it you want in your life and determine the price to get it. Your price could be the book you should read and the effort you should put into succeeding.

I strongly believe that success is a learnable skill. Either you can learn by yourself or from others. Success is not a skill we all are born with; we learn everything here throughout our journey of life. This skill is neither easy nor hard. That is why famous businessman Henry Ford once said, if you think you can or you cannot, in both ways you are right. Which one do you want to choose? The power of choice is in your hands. Between these two options, if I need to choose, I will always choose "I can" and go for it. If I lose the battle sometimes, I will stand up again, retry it and utilize my past battle as a learning process to overcome the obstacles I am facing in the present. So, I never want to quit the journey I choose. Rather, I will go till the road ends. For me, it's an adventure and learning process and experiment that gives me a lot of knowledge and experiences that always please me. There are two types of success; one is personal success, and the other is organizational success. After you achieve personal success, you go and connect with the organization of your choice. You need to work for the success of the organization. So, I will share both based on my understanding and experiences throughout my life journey.

Personal success is mostly related to personal habits and choices we make during our life journey. Healthy and successful habits create a healthy and successful life. Making a successful habit is challenging and needs discipline and commitment in everyday life. You need to watch and observe your behaviour patterns yourself. Even if sometimes you are off track, pull yourself back on track; it is normal. Consistent trying and self-discipline are required to cultivate successful habits. Once the habit is formed, you can focus completely on the task at hand and no one can stop you from reaching your target. It means if you can focus and you see only your target, there is a higher chance to hit the target. If you lose focus, you may miss the target. When I studied, many success- related books said that you need to be motivated to achieve success. But the reality is motivation does not last longer just like a bath. You have a morning bath, but after you go to the office, you get dirty again, and you need to take another bath before going to bed (McGrath 2005). In reality, sometimes we forget our goal and target and seek motivation after motivation and at the end of the day, we lose sight of the target. So, we needed the inner motivation rather than outer motivation; that is the purpose. If you have higher purpose and reason, you do not need outer motivation. There is inside you the higher purpose which can be a great motivator that can wake you up and help you, even in the difficulties. The reason to do something and the reason to achieve something is always stronger than any other motivation.

To achieve personal success greatly, you need to have a strong desire that was chosen by yourself. You may need to question; how do you find whether the desire is yours or not? The answer is if this is a deep-rooted desire, it controls your mind. Your thought will be closely related to your desire. For example, if you fall deeply in love with someone, your thoughts will be related to love of that person. The love of that person controls the mind, and according to the thought process, you will do activities. According to your activities, the results ultimately come to you. That means unless you desire excellent results you will not achieve excellent results. So, if you start the journey, it will be important to desire excellency. That desire develops the excellent thought process that leads to excellent action and ultimately gives you excellent results. Everyone has their own personal Mount Everest to conquer (Woodbury & De Ora 2008). While climbing Mount Everest, sometimes the weather gives you a challenge and some even die despite their guide and expedition management. Like the challenge of climbing Mount Everest, there are challenges in your Bachelor of Nursing clinical placement as well because you might get a tough and challenging facilitator. Some students might be lucky because they get a good, caring and supportive facilitator. They may support you and help you to achieve excellent results. Some may face very challenging ones, and they may even make you fail in the subjects. It's a reality I am talking about. The outcome is not in our hands. The only thing in our hands is we can get stronger, smarter and powerful enough to handle their pressure. The only thing that matters in your life is whether you became skilful or not. Pass and fail is temporary. It comes and goes in life. Even if you fail, its temporary not permanent. You have the opportunity to pass in the next attempt. If you learned the lesson in life and became experienced that ultimately gives you the joy in the long run while perusing your career goal. I can bet with anyone that you all have the power to accomplish your desire and dreams no matter what and how difficult it is. The power of choice is in your hands and ultimately only in your hands to accomplish anything you want and to make the difference in your life and others' lives.

The two purposes of writing this book are to make you aware of the pitfalls in the clinical placements and how to overcome those obstacles and achieve excellent results. Another one is to help your new graduate nursing program job interview to attain excellent results. I have written in the practical examples how theory can be implemented in a practical setting. How do you get excellent results in the interview? The main target is to achieve success in the interview and enhance learning by applying theory into practice. For that reason, I have identified what to focus on in the interview preparation process and shared some important questions which my friends and I encountered in the job interview. I have put forward all the questions types with answers as well as possible to make you successful in the new graduate nursing interview. The nursing role and clinical questions which are scenario-based questions are universally acknowledged and can be utilized in the nursing interview as well as clinical practice. Also, in the interview preparation I have mentioned a method that can be useful to achieve good results in any job interview. I utilized the technique, and I secured the new graduate nursing job at the hospital in Sydney, Australia. In fact, I put a lot of effort in this book to prepare the answers than I actually prepared for my own interview. This means the questions and the answers I prepared are really powerful. If someone, asked to buy this book permanently, in fact, I could not sell it no matter what the price they offered. To prepare this book, I compiled thousands of hours of writing, studying and gaining clinical experiences. The whole purpose of writing this book is to make you successful. I admired the philosophy of Buddha. He himself was the son of a king more than 2600 hundred years ago. Despite all the palace's facility and luxurious life, he went to the jungle alone and visited many places in search of wisdom to remove sorrows from the life of human beings in those ancient days. After 7 years of meditation, he got enlightenment, and he visited many places to share the wisdom and to remove sorrow permanently from the life of human beings. His three words always hit me: APPO DEEPO BHAWA. That means in English to be a lamp unto yourself. I only can light the others and remove the darkness if I became the lamp myself. I have been through difficulties in clinical placement; yet, I learned to be successful. I applied clinical skills I learnt in the clinical placement and in a job interview and achieved success. That is why I want to share this as much as possible so my experience and ideas I experimented with can benefit others.

If you read this book before you attend the clinical placement, it will guide you through your journey. This book's role is to work like Tanging Norge Sherpa who was appointed by Sir Edmund Hillary to support and guide him to climb Mount Everest successfully. So, your personal Mount Everest journey begins at the clinical placement (base camp of Everest) to Everest's summit when you successfully secure the new graduate nursing position at a hospital. This is the whole journey. One question that arises is why did Sir Edmund Hillary appoint Tanging Norge Sherpa as a guide? In life, whether we climb Mount Everest or do clinical placement, on the road we all have blind spots. The problem is we don't always know what they are. We should bear in mind that these blind spots exist and the way to reveal and eliminate them is to open your mind to new solutions and new ideas (Woodbury & De Ora 2008). In this situation, you may need assistance and guidance. The reason in writing this book is to guide you throughout the process to climb your own Mount Everest to reach your career goal.

Like Sir Edmund Hillary recruited the most experienced Sherpa Tanging Norgay to assist him, you also can take help from this book to achieve your career goal successfully. Like Norgay knew the landscape immediately, I know its exact landscape because I have been through this. Where inexperienced eyes would see a mountain of difficulty, Norgay saw a clear path while climbing Mount Everest. He could identify the dangers and manage the risks. Finally, he guided mountaineers to the summit and brought them safely back to the camp (Woodbury & De Ora 2008). Like Tanging Norgay Sherpa, this book will guide and assist you through your clinical placement and help you to secure a new graduate nursing program in the hospital successfully. Are you ready for the journey? Here is some evidence of additional comment given to me by my clinical facilitator in my last clinical placement. I would like to thank and acknowledge her guidance to my last PEP. I would also like to thank her for the comments she made. These comments inspired me so much while continuing the writing and finishing this book for upcoming students. I am fully committed to implementing all the clinical skills I learnt to achieve health and well-being for the patient.

Mohan Sangraula

Additional Comments

Mohan has demonstrated significant leap in his confidence level and clinical reasoning in the last few weeks of this 8 week long placement. He managed to incorporate all the suggested feedback and displayed ability to remain proactive and engaged in many aspects of nursing care provision. He was able to provide comprehensive, holistic, safe & competent care to patients under his care. He actively sought learning opportunities as well as able to identify his own limitations. He adhered to all components and domains of ANMC standards throughout this placement. He is a safe and competent practitioner and would make a devoted, diligent and sincere nurse. Well done!

Clinical Facilitator name:	Initial:	Signature:	Date:
USHMA RAYAMAJHI	UR	*[signature]*	21/01/16

7

Student: **Mohan Sangraula** i.d: **180258**   Review a, b, c, (d,)(circle)

BN competency Assessment Tool (PEP 4/5)   **18/01/2016**   use ✔

Professional Practice	I	S	A	M	D
1. Practises in accordance with legislation affecting nursing practice and health care	✓				
2. Practises within a professional and ethical framework	✓				
Critical Thinking and Analysis	✓				
3. Practises with an evidence based framework	✓				
4. Participates in ongoing professional development of self and others	✓				
Provision and Coordination of Care	✓				
5. Conducts a comprehensive and systematic nursing assessment	✓				
6. Plans nursing care with individuals/groups, significant others and interdisciplinary health care teams	✓				
7. Provides comprehensive safe and effective evidence based care to achieve individual/group health outcomes	✓				
8. Evaluates progress towards expected health outcomes in consultation with individuals/groups and the healthcare team	✓				
Collaborative and Therapeutic Practice	✓				
9. Establishes, maintains and appropriately concludes therapeutic relationships	✓				
10. Collaborates with the interdisciplinary health care team to provide comprehensive nursing care	✓				

Independent:	I	Refers to being safe and knowledgeable; proficient and coordinated and appropriately confident and timely. Does not require supporting cues.
Supervised:	S	Refers to being safe & knowledgeable; efficient & coordinated; displays some confidence and undertakes activities within a reasonably timely manner. Requires occasional supporting cues.
Assisted:	A	Refers to being safe and knowledgeable most of the time; skillful in parts however is inefficient with some skill areas; takes longer than would be expected to complete the task. Requires frequent verbal and some physical cues.
Marginal:	M	Refers to being safe when closely supervised and supported; unskilled and inefficient; uses excess energy and takes a prolonged time period. Continuous verbal and physical cues.
Dependent:	D	Refers to concerns about being unsafe and being unable to demonstrate behaviour or articulate intention; lacking in confidence, coordination and efficiency. Continuous verbal and physical cues/interventions necessary.

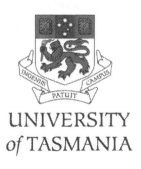

UNIVERSITY
of TASMANIA

In accordance with the Rules of the University

Mohan Sangraula

has this day been admitted to the degree of

Bachelor of Nursing

*in evidence of which this certificate is issued
under the Seal of the University*

CHANCELLOR

VICE-CHANCELLOR

Dated this twenty sixth day of April 2016
Award number: 56339

ORGANIZATIONAL SUCCESS

In any organisation, a group of people work together to achieve the organizational goal. Employees who work in the organization play a vital role in its success. That is why it is significant to develop the habit of a sense of urgency; this habit is possessing by only 2 percent of the population. Two percent of the population do things fast, and two percent of the population have a bias for action. In Tom Peters' wonderful book, *In Search of Excellence,* he says that all great and excellent companies have a bias of action. All the others who are not committed to being excellent do the things when they feel like doing them. He gave the example of IBM. If someone calls them for a problem or information, they cannot let you off the phone. In two minutes they will sort it out. So, get the habit and reputation for doing things fast. To put the employee on track to success in any company is first its ability to set priorities to determine what is relevant and what is irrelevant and number two is a sense of urgency. In any health care setting, setting priorities and utilizing a sense of urgency to attain the patient concern fast can save a lot of lives and promote quality care. So, develop the habit of prioritizing the care of patients and a sense of urgency to bring excellent results in your health care setting.

HOW TO SUCCEED IN CHALLENGING BACHELOR OF NURSING CLINICAL PLACEMENT?

Every individual responds differently to challenging situation throughout their clinical journey. Some challenges are very important for the student to learn and respond to correctly in the clinical environment. It is my opinion that when the challenge comes to my life I always remember the story about the creation of diamonds. The formation of natural diamonds occurs because of very high temperature and pressures. It means that challenge and pressures are good if it has a constructive purpose. Every individual has a different tolerance of pressure and challenges. Thus, it depends upon on how you handle the situation and what your perception is. Therefore, if you encounter challenges in your clinical placement please take it as a lesson, make your mind at peace and always focus on the learning aspect of the situation. This is in fact a great moment for the student as you are going to get practical learning skills which you are going to implement in your whole career. In this chapter I have highlighted some skills which are based on my knowledge and experiences for your benefit to succeed. These are the following skills.

Be confident

You need to be confident while you answer the questions of your Facilitator and Preceptors. Please think that they are also a human being like you. Joel Osteen America's famous Bible preacher said that confidence is an important ingredient to succeed in life. To be a confident you need to always tell to yourself, I am confident. To be a confident, you should put your shoulder back, hold your head up high, walk confidently, talk confidently, think confidently and act confidently. People are going to treat you the way you present yourself. While you talk, look at the person eyes confidently, not arrogantly and present yourself well. Believe that you are not less than anybody else. Feel strong and secured, even if you do not feel confident, just act confidently. In these moments, you feel generally better about yourself. The more you do it, the more you will feel good about yourself and finally you will become the confident person you need to be. It is the requirement of Bachelor of Nursing competency assessment. You can check in your BN competency tool. It has clearly mentioned.

Independent I – Refers to being safe and knowledgeable; proficient and coordinated and **appropriately confident and timely.** Does not require supporting cues.

Therefore, if you are aiming to achieve this "Independent" quality in your clinical placement please do not forget to talk confidently, walk confidently, think confidently and act confidently. Please present yourself as good as possible.

Personal Hygiene

When you get up from sleep in the morning, at first your body is in lethargy. To remove the lethargy from the body, you may need to do light exercises for a few minutes and have a shower.

It only takes you a few minutes and makes you feel energetic the whole day, you feel fit and fresh. That also helps to boost your confidence level in the clinical placement. People like people who are fit, fresh and energetic.

Commit to do safe practices

To commit to do safe practices daily in the clinical placement, you need to be aware of these safe practices. Your Facilitator is always observing directly or indirectly the following safe practices.

- Wear a dress recommend by the University and student name badge.
- Introduce yourself to the patient and your role and always take consent before doing anything to the patient.
- While doing clinical placement please always observe whether the patient has arm band or not. If he or she has not had an arm band, you need to talk to the preceptor and organize arm band for safety reasons.
- Before giving the medication check whether the patient has any known allergies or not. You can check in the medication chart in the ADR (allergies and adverse reaction) section at the top left side of the medication chart. Patient needs to wear a red arm band if they have allergies.
- If you are handling cytotoxic patient or cytotoxic waste, please use and wear cytotoxic personal protective equipment.
- Infection control- wear appropriate personal protective equipment.
- Hand Hygiene (know and apply five moments of hand hygiene).
- Use alcohol based hand rub as required for infection control reason.
- Please follow five rights (right patient, right medication, right time, right dose and right route) and documentation.

Indication

Student generally focus on the six rights for the medication administration. Sometimes student get confused if the facilitator asks suddenly why the patient is having for example, Aspirin. He may forget to look in the indication section in the medication chart to know the answer. You may find the answer there easily if you have practiced to look there before giving the medication. In the indication section, the doctor always writes the indication of the medication for example you may find in the indication section a DVT for Aspirin, Oedema for Furosemide. If your facilitator is a challenging type, he or she may ask you further questions: Which drugs class is Aspirin in? You need to tell him/her during situation that Aspirin is an Antiplatelet agent. He/she may further challenge you what does it do? You need to tell him/her the Antiplatelet agents which inhibit this unwanted thrombus formation by decreasing platelet aggregation. He/she may further challenge you what thrombus means? You need to tell him/her a blood clot has formed within the vascular system that may prevent blood flow.

The reason for writing this is to make you aware that you need to get into the habit of looking at the indication section so that you can answer any question your facilitator or preceptor may have. If you practice to look at the indication section including the six rights, you can confidently administer the medication and that creates a sense of accomplishment for yourself. If you do not know some of the medications, you need to look at MIMS and try to look at specific aspects of the drug for example, Mechanism of action, the adverse effect and the drug class.

Respect your Clinical Facilitator

Respect your Clinical Facilitator and preceptor, they deserve your respect because they are transferring their skills and knowledge. Give them the world class respect so that they feel like they want to transfer all the skills they have. You need to be more clear that your clinical result is fully controlled by the clinical facilitator. So, do not involve in any unnecessary arguments. You just need to follow their guidance, listen attentively what they say and follow their instruction and assignment deadlines and focus only in learning. There is no other option left.

Quick reference guide for abbreviations and medical terminology

Find out or ask in your allocated ward if they have reference guide for abbreviation and medical terminology. Medical officer and other health care teams frequently writes in abbreviations in their writing. For example,

AAA= abdominal aortic aneurysm
AX= assessment
AXR= Abdominal X-ray
BIBA=brought in by ambulance
BX= Biopsy
CXR= chest X-ray
AB's= Antibiotics
/24= indicating hours
/7= indicating days
/52= indicating weeks
/12= indicating months
Wt.= weight
A= Assist
I= independent

There are many more abbreviations used. So, search online or find in the ward frequently used medical abbreviation to improve your learning and understanding.

How to answer the Facilitator's questions and succeed?

Whenever you encounter some new equipment in your placement area, you need to ask three questions to know the answer for example, what is it called? what does it do? and where does it attach, or insert? For example, I have a patient who has an intercostal catheter (ICC), in that case if my facilitator asks me: what is it called? My answer should be intercostal catheter (ICC). He might ask me, what does it do? I need to reply him ICC helps drainage air and fluids from the lungs. He may ask again which parts of the lungs; at this situation, I need to answer the actual space for example plural space. So, ask your preceptor or research yourself to find the answer whenever you encounter with a new equipment or procedure to answer the Facilitator's questions successfully.

Whenever you encounter a new procedure or a new disease, for example the procedure for the patient completed was second stage of oesophagoctomy. Oesophagoctomy means the removal of the oesophagus, but you may find difficulty for understanding what the second stage means, it can either be a cancer stage or an operative stage. You may ask the preceptor to know about which stage it is. If they could not answer, you may ask the doctor who has completed the procedure. They usually visit the patient in the ward and at that time you can politely ask them questions you have relating to either of the procedures. They will tell you the exact procedure. In the second stage of oesophagoctomy represents the operative stage not the cancer stage for that condition. If you have the right answer, it will be easier to answer the questions asked by the facilitator.

Mt. Everest Mountaineering Versus Clinical Placement

You need to strive for the best and prepare for the worst. When mountaineers go to successfully climb a mountain, they have a guide, they have an expedition plan, safety plan, oxygen, medicine and food. They have all the necessary equipment someone needs to climb that mountain. While they are climbing the mountains, suddenly the weather may change and they may face the challenge of snow fall, snow storm and avalanche. It may seem impossible to go ahead. In this type of situation, if they move ahead, they may die because mountain or nature's destructive emotion (snow fall, snow storm and avalanche) are so high. In this type of situation climbers' priority should be their safety. If they survive, they can climb many more mountains successfully. At this type of situation, they need to use their intelligence and brain power to survive not emotions or rigidity. Emotions are so attached with the result or outcome and victory. They should use their brain and intelligence not the emotion to survive, human emotions are as destructible as like mountains or natures emotions for example snow storm or avalanche. It is impossible to stop the natures emotions. The climbers have the choices to move ahead or stop, they can let go their emotions of victory and use their brain and intelligence to survive. Alike this, in your clinical expedition, if you are challenged by your facilitator and you feel that it's impossible to go ahead or move ahead. I cannot tell you exactly what you should do at this type of situation but If I were in your position I would let go my destructive emotions. Alike experienced mountaineers do, stop the challenging journey for a while, think and analyses the situation and I would follow the brain and human intelligence instead of negative emotion to survive and thrive in the future. We as a human being, have a great power which is the power of choice. We can choose what to do and choices are limitless. I believe if you understand the power of your brain's intelligence and power of your choices, you can overcome any obstacle life throws on you.

You can solve any difficult problem or situation no matter how difficult it may be. Emotions are energy just like electricity you can use it to do positive work for example, currents can be used to light the electric bulb or it can be used for the lift in the house or building and current also can kill the person if he touches it with his bare hand. You cannot control your emotion but the good thing is you can direct it in a positive direction or use it to do the positive meaning full work. Always focus on the learning aspect of any difficult situation and from there you may prosper. I would also like to recommend to use your intelligence power in the challenging situation to survive and thrive in the future.

Be flexible

In the very famous classic book Toa The Ching written by Lao Tzu tell us about the way of living. Toa The Ching means way of living. In chapter no. 76, it has written that "when he is born man is soft and weak. In death, he becomes stiff and hard. Truly what is stiff and hard is a companion of death and what is soft and weak is companion of life". So, if you want to be alive or survive, you need to be flexible. Flexible not only in terms of our body but in terms of our mind, in terms of our thinking and belief. Let's be ready to change.

There is always a next time

Life is beautiful and let's be ready to change. There is always a next day, next event, next opportunity waiting for all of us. If we survive there are many mountains waiting for us to climb. We certainly can climb it, when the weather is clear, pleasant, bright and favorable. There are many more pleasant and favorable weathers welcoming us. When you go through the difficulty, always turn towards the bright side and new possibilities for example it may be acquiring a new habit or new skills.

Reverse thinking

Famous philosopher and mind technologist of Nepal Dr. Yogi Bikashanandha once said in an interview that whenever something bad happens, you need to instantly think about what was the good about this incident. For example, you slipped on the corridor in your work place and your leg fractured. It's a bad incident, everybody knows it. If you take it as a bad incident and worry too much about your leg, it can cause a negative state of mind such as depression. Instead of worrying about your leg, you need to search what is good about it. The good thing may be, you will get compensation from your work for two months. You do get bed rest for two months. At this period, you can have a complete rest, listening music, read a book you like, many friend will visit to you and you might get lots of wishes. John McGrath famous real-estate agent of Australia mentioned in his book You INC that whenever he encounters some problem and difficulties, he always looks for the gift hiding inside the problem. In business man's life, every day new problems comes. The way of overcoming that is look for the positive side of any bad incident or situation. That is how they are surviving and thriving.

Regular exercise and sleep well

Make a habit of regular exercise at least 20 minutes. Without exercise human being, cannot be healthy physically and psychologically. Scientists have found that while you do exercise body releases endorphin that automatically makes you happy. So, every day you need to do it, if you want to be happy and energetic. That can be anything for example, running, cycling, swimming and dancing. After any exercise, your body needs to rest adequately. If you sleep deeply for example, 7 to 9 hours a day, it makes your mood good, memory and brain power increases and increases the learning capacity. So, to be in deep sleep zone, you may need to use a dark curtain in your bedroom because light can disturb your sleep. Sleep is very important because our mind will clean in the deep sleep just like to remove junk and virus, we need to reformat the computer. Deep sleep will reformat our mind. We need to have a good deep sleep to make our mind and body healthy. That is why in English there is a saying 'sleep and grow'.

YATHA DRISHTI TATHA SRISTI

In thousands of years ago in Vedas it was mentioned '**Yatha Drishti Tatha Sristi**'. These words are extremely powerful and will remain relevant to human life forever. It means that how you see the world, the world will appear to you in the same way. In other words, Drishti means our sight and Sristi means creation. Whatever our vision is accordingly that is how the whole world appears to us. To make a good thing happen you need to look at positive side. For example, three friends went to visit to see the sea side. The first one is enjoying by looking at the sea and enjoying the cool breeze of the sea. The second friend is watching the naked women. He is not looking at the sea and feeling the breeze of the wind means he misses the enjoyment of the sea. The third friend is neither looking at naked woman nor the sea, he is thinking about his ex-girlfriend and still thinking that why she had left him and he is also missing the enjoyment of the sea. The same situation or circumstances they have right now means they are near the sea side but they are thinking and looking at differently despite the same situation. Their vision is different such a way their creation is different. When your Drishti (vision) change than only the Sristi (creation) will change. So always see good, listen good and speak good. That certainly can bring positive changes in your life. There is no other option left. When you light in the darkness, it automatically removes darkness. Whenever you go towards the light the darkness will disappear.

Similarly, knowledge, wisdom and skills development removes all the negativity and skills lacking in the clinical setting as well.

While you are heading to do your PEP, often, the student neglects their personal health and well-being. Health is the most important aspect and should be prioritised. If you maintain your health, it can keep you fit for the work and studies as well.

So, drink plenty of water and maintain hydration at all times. For the PEP and studies, you may need a lot of energy, and I believe sources of energy come from mainly three things: food, positive thinking, and meditation.

Food

The brain controls the body. So, while the brain is challenged by hectic work in the PEP and assignments it might need fuel to stay focused and absorb what you actually learnt. Milk and yogurt (low-fat dairy products) are packed with B vitamins and protein that may help you work efficiently and help you to concentrate. It also has vitamin D which also supports brain health. Having oats in the breakfast which has whole grain that you digest gives your brain and body steady energy. Salmon is one of the good sources of omega -3 fatty acids, healthy fats that are good for the brain. You can have walnuts, plenty of green vegetables and all kinds of fruits which also supports brain health as well as the body (Dementia Collaborative Research centre (DCRC) 2014).

Positive Thinking

In real life, it's true that despite our positive thinking, we may sometimes be unsuccessful. Sometimes, we might not get the result we wanted. It's not always true that if I think positive, positive thing always happens to me. If someone has this type of belief, unfortunately, this is not very true. It is just a superstition. I like the saying of the Lord Krishna in the book Gita, positive thinking is not about expecting the best to happen always in your favour. It's about accepting that whatever happens, happens for the best. This type of positive thinking is reality-based and empowers you to make positive change. Even if you lose the battle sometimes, this type of thinking ultimately makes you successful. This type of positive thinking gives you energy, and you will not be scared by failure. You always can learn from your failure. History shows how failure is essential to all achievement, that great success is always accompanied by great failure (Staples 1991). Thomas Edison had to discover over ten thousand ways a light bulb would not work before he discovered the one way it would (Staples 1991). He had a very different attitude toward his work. He looked upon each unsuccessful attempt not as a failure but as a success, a success that took him one step closer to his ultimate goal (Staples 1991). He kept his focus firmly on the goal he was striving for and was willing to do whatever was necessary to reach it. It worked for him. He was the most prolific inventor in modern history, with 1,097 devices patented in his name (Staples 1991).

Meditation

Mediation also supports and develops focus and concentration power. It also brings self-containment and causeless happiness to your life. There are a lot of techniques to do meditation, but I actually prefer the technique which lord Krishna had taught to Arjun in Mahabharata approximately 5 thousand years ago which was written in Gita. To do this type of meditation, you need to sit in a quiet place in a comfortable posture. Concentrate in between the two eyebrows for a while. If you have any thought in your mind, you need to empty it, or you can concentrate "0" on that space. After a while, you will become thoughtless. Then concentrate on breathing slowly in and out and feel it.

Concentrating on breathing is a tool which connects your mind and body. Then the joy you feel in your mind comes to your body, and you will become thoughtless, and you will feel happy. Lord Buddha tells about when you slowly enter your body and observe the starting point of any thought inside your body. In this way, while you observe, you will become thoughtless. Buddha gave it the name middle point '0 space' and told us to focus on it to get happiness. It means, be in the present moment and be the observer and that makes you thoughtless and happy. I believe meditation is the journey of the internal to bring joy and true happiness in life. In that way, you can observe your thought and choose your thoughts to your benefit. That gives you control of everything, for example, anger, any hatred, and anything. Buddha said it is the way of enlightenment. Be the observer of self and live in the present moment. It all depends on your level of practice and your level of focus. The more you practice, the more you get happiness and self-control. The happiness you will get from meditation is priceless and cannot to be compared to any degree, wealth, power, and any earthly accomplishment. Buddha clearly stated after his 7-year search for happiness; happiness is a choice, not a result. Nothing will make you happy until you choose to be happy. No person will make you happy unless you decide to be happy. Your happiness will not come to you. It can only come from you. You need to search happiness inside you, and the way is through meditation. I am practicing it daily 5, 10 or 20 minutes whenever it's possible for me. You can also practice if you want joy and happiness in your life. It all depends on you. Lord Buddha said that the first step you need to take; then it will pull you towards joy and happiness.

Awareness and observation skill

To increase awareness and observation skill, you need to develop total focus and concentration skill. For that, you need to pay attention to the present moment. You should not be thinking about the past and the future. In regards to both the past and the future, you don't have any control at the moment. It means wherever you are, be there. Awareness is also called the light. When you are aware you develop control which means you can completely take control of any situation. It's a skill and highly needed to be successful in any field. I will share one example; we were altogether six students and had given a math calculation test. We needed to secure 100% to pass the test and if you failed you needed to make another attempt but needed 100%. It was the requirement of CNA 322 professional practice PEP. We were all given the test; there were 10 questions. We needed to complete that test in half an hour. We all completed it and handed over to the facilitator. When the result came, what happened was I passed the test on the first attempt and the facilitator congratulated me. She said that you are the only one who passed the test. The other 5 students missed the same easy question. They all could not see one question which was at the bottom of the second page. The question they all missed was very easy too. Due to lack of awareness and observation skill, they missed the question. At that time, I was practicing awareness and observation skill, so I checked every question thoroughly so that I could be able to do the test successfully. So, I am practiceing it and committed to do life long. If you want, you can practice too. You cannot buy or borrow this skill. You need to practice it every day by paying attention at the present moment. You can watch the English movie *Peaceful Warrior* by Dan Millman. If you watch this movie, you will understand what I am actually talking about. This is one of my favourite movies I have ever watched. It's all about how important it is to live in the present moment and every moment is significant in life and how to cultivate happiness in life by focusing on the journey of the life instead of a destination. But most of us always focus towards the destination and miss the real experience of the life journey. By the time we reach the destination, the destination cannot give any happiness and we are simply fed up with that and our expectations will not be met. There will not be anything we are truly searching for. What's going on around you, any important event or situation is very significant. The present moment you lost cannot be brought back. It means that you need to give 100% at the present moment so that your mind focuses on the task you are doing rather than the past and future situation which does not matter to you. So, remember to be aware and observant to focus at the present moment.

Be Thankful

One of the bitter truths is that power generates ego inside the person. Anger comes from ego-based beliefs of being right and knowing better than someone else. You may encounter various types of personality in the PEP; it is normal. You just need to be thankful to them and grateful for the learning opportunity. We cannot change other people's attitudes. You need to get ready to learn from the good preceptor and the challenging one as well. Even if sometimes you could not answer the questions they asked, you would need to politely tell them, you are unsure about the answer at the moment. You will research it and explain to them after. In this type of situation, you need to do research and make sure you tell them in detail later. This shows that you are committed to learning and able to ensure research-based practice. So always be thankful to them for their efforts to transfer their skills to you. Always discuss your matters only to the concerned person. Always take feedback from them and be thankful for their valued feedback. Never make negative personal comments to anyone. We are all responsible for creating a fabulous learning environment for ourselves and others.

How to excel in PEP and successfully complete

Ask your facilitator the objectives of the PEP and its requirement. Generally, on the first day of the PEP, your facilitator will give an orientation regarding the PEP objectives, requirement, and your responsibility. You need to be more clear about your job responsibility and your limitations. What you can do and what you should not do.

Shift Planner and hand over helper sheet

I am explaining here about the third-year PEP. If you understand, it may cover all your PEP needs. First, you need to have a shift planner to plan your day and the other is the handover helper sheet. You can download and keep the print with you so that you can use it for PEP. These are the tools you need to use from the beginning of the shift to the end of the shift. In the shift planner, you need to write in every hour what care you need to deliver to your patients. The shift planner will remind you of care delivery, priority and time. To fill the shift planner, you collect the important information from the daily care plan, the doctor's note, and medication charts. In the handover sheet, you can write what care you did during your shift and any care needs to be done in the other shift as per the doctor's order and nursing care plan. If you use these two tools and write the information there, you can easily explain to your preceptor and facilitator. Update your shift planner and handover helper as per the changes in your shift. I am sure your facilitator and preceptor will be impressed, if you followed it at all times and you have all the information in your hand as well. Notes and charts are most of the time carried and used by other health care teams as well. So, if you have information written in the shift planner and handover helper, you can easily answer the questions of the preceptor and the facilitator when they ask you, and you can provide care delivery to the patients in a timely manner.

Time management table sheet

Bed Number	0800	0900	1000	1100	1200	1300	1400	1500

Handover Helper sheet

Bed Number	Name Age Doctor/ Team	Reason for admission/ Diagnosis	Relevant Medical History	Alert/ Oriented/ Mobility Needs Continence IDC/SPC	Relevant Dietary needs	IVT/FBC Special meds and Charts	Procedure and Consults	Plans For discharge

Important Drug Calculation Formulas

These are the important medication calculation formulas you may need to know before the medication administration. So, practice well at home and remember to follow the formulas. The formulas are the tools to calculate the drugs accurately, and that ensures patient safety.

Drug Calculation Formulas

Conversions
milligrams to grams = mg divided by 1000   e.g. 1000 mg = 1 g

grams to milligrams = g x 1000   e.g. 1 g = 1000 mg

Amount required =   **dose required** x volume
                                   stock strength

e.g.   dose require = 2g, stock strength = 1g per tab

    = $\frac{2}{1}$ x 1 = 2 tabs

e.g.   dose required = 5g, stock strength = 10g per 5 ml

             $\frac{5}{10}$ x 5 = 2.5 ml

$\frac{volume}{time}$ e.g. 1000mls to be infused over 4 hours = $\frac{1000}{4}$ = 250 mls/ hr

$\frac{volume \times 60}{time (min)}$ e.g. 100mls over 20 min = $\frac{100}{20}$ x 60 = 300mls/hr

$\frac{volume}{time}$ x $\frac{drip factor}{60}$ (macro = 20 dpm, micro = 60 dpm)

e.g.   1000mls to be infused over 10 hrs via macro drip

       $\frac{1000}{10}$ x $\frac{20}{60}$ = 33.333dpm = 33 dpm

mg x kg (milligrams per kilogram)   e.g. 2 mg x 20 kg = 40mg

Communication skill

Active listening is required to absorb the information and process it for its implementation. Focus in the present moment helps us to develop listening skills to concentrate on the task at hand. If you have not quite caught the information, you needed to ask for clarification and request to repeat it. Verbal speaking is also important in nursing. You need to hand over the information clearly to the next shift, interact with a multidisciplinary team and with the patient. It is required to speak clearly and politely to everybody; otherwise, miscommunication happens. Always remember and make sure your information is understood by the listener or receiver. Writing in clear, understandable and legible handwriting is required to make the other health care teams able to understand your communication. Always remember that your writing represents you and it shows your level of communication. It is also a legal document so extra care and attention should be given to avoid communication misfires. Many health care officers and nursing staff members ignore this which results in difficulty to understand their writing and it's also time-consuming to read their writing. For example, once I was reading a doctor's plan of care for the day. His handwriting was unclear, and I asked my preceptor, and she was also unsure about the information. She said, "I presumed that it should be this". The doctor's handwriting was not clear, and this caused a delay in trying to understand his writing and to act for the treatment processes. So, while I start to write my progress notes, I remember this incident and consciously decide to write clear, legible and understandable progress notes to make understanding my writing easy to other health care teams. You can do the same, if you wish. It can bring a change that helps others and saves their time as well. You just need to ask one question before writing: Will my writing be understandable to others? You just need to write carefully and consciously. I believe anyone can do that and make the difference.

Progress note sample

Date: 04/04/2016, 1400 pm

Pt is alert and at times confused. Vital signs stable a febrile. Medications are given to pt as charted. Pt is in MScontin BD and given to the patient as charted with good effect. Nil breakthrough required during AM shift. Assisted to prepare his meals and pt is tolerating his diet and fluids. Pt remains high risk of falls. Assistance requires + 1 nurse for mobility and personal care. Skin intact, Uri dome in situ and draining well. Random BSL before -lunch time was 6.6 mmol. Bowel open in this AM shift. Plan- awaiting bed in 6 west rehab. Written by UTAS Student Nurse Mohan Sangraula, Preceptor signature is required.

Above is a sample of progress note writing which I learned during PEP. This is one of the ways to write progress notes. Your preceptor will guide you. Generally, in progress notes, we write what we actually did to our patient during our shift, the current situation and what the plan is.

Understanding of the Patient whole situation

Generally, the patient has a medical history, presenting problem and reason to admit to the hospital. To find out the presenting problem, the medical diagnosis process begins. For that reason, the doctor can send him/her for various tests (e.g., blood test, x-ray, ultrasound, echo, biopsy).As per the requirement, the doctor sends the patient for the test. By analysing the prognosis of a disease or presenting problem and by analysing various tests, the doctor finalizes their diagnosis. After that, the patient's treatment process begins. After the treatment, discharge comes into effect and some patients discharge to home and some discharge to aged care nursing and rehab. As per the interdisciplinary teams' decision, the patient will be discharged. We need to understand why the patient is in hospital? What test needs to be done for him? What are the medications and treatment processes for him? Where is he going after the treatment? These are the questions you need to keep in mind for the patient you are looking after and find the information from the handover, doctor's note, progress note and care plan and execute them as per the order. Always remember you need to be supervised by the preceptor at all times and never cross the professional boundary.

Use of MIMS

If you are not sure about any medication, you should not give it to the patient. You first need to look into the MIMS. MIMS can be available in the format of a book and online as well. Before giving the medication to the patient, if I am not sure about medication, I always view the hospital's reference viewer available in the hospital's Internet. I constantly referred to the online MIMS, drug guidebook. For example, if I had to look for the information about Ramipril (medicine name) In online MIMS, I used the MIMS service provided by the clinical information access portal (CIAP) which was available through hospital's Internet service. For example, I received this information for Ramipril (medicine).

Use: Hypertension, post – MI, heart failure

Drug class: ACE inhibitor, antihypertensive agents

Common adverse reactions: Hypotension, persistent dry cough, renal impairment and hyperkalaemia (Tiziani 2010).

Before giving this medication to the patient, I always considered checking a patient's blood pressure. If the patient was hypotensive, I delayed the medication until the blood pressure improved (as supervised and permission from my preceptor).

Use of Australian Injectable drugs handbook (AIDH)

You can use it as a book, or you can look at in online. I used the book as well as the online copy. To view online, I used the AIDH service provided by CIAP which was available through hospital's Internet service. For example, the medication order for the patient I was looking after was Caftrixone 1 gram (surgical prophylaxis) via intravenous (IV). At this situation, I need to go online to the Australian injectable drugs handbook (AIDH). I looked at the information about the method of preparation and fluid compatibility. For IV route, I prepared this drug with 1 gram with 10 ml of water (AIDH).

Administration: Inject doses up to 1 gram over 2 to 4 minutes through IV line (AIDH). These are the ways to find information regarding drugs and their safe administration practices in clinical settings. If you follow it, you will be able to administer the medication safely to the patient. Always remember patient safety comes first.

Important Nursing Tools

Five Rights

The primary role of the Australian Health Practitioner Regulatory Agency (AHPRA) is to protect the public (NMBA 2006). As a student nurse while I was practicing in the hospital environment my primary role was to do practice safely and make sure the safety of the patient was highly maintained. For the safety of the patient, as a nurse I used some of the nursing clinical tools which do not only help to bring safety of the patient, it also brought the best health outcome to the patient. The first nursing clinical tool I used was five rights of medication administration. Before administering the medications for the safety of the patient, I confirmed and checked the five rights: the right patient, the right drug, the right dose, the right route and the right time. I also checked whether the patient has any known allergy history and the expiry of the medication to be used. I documented and signed with my preceptor in every shift I worked. This is considered one of the safest practices in nursing for medication administration (Levitt-Jones et al. 2009).

Clinical Reasoning Cycle (Reflection)

Secondly, I used the clinical reasoning cycle to conduct the comprehensive nursing assessment. It is considered in nursing as a clinical decision-making tool, to achieve the best and safe health outcome for the patient. While doing a comprehensive nursing assessment, I followed these eight crucial steps for the safety of the patient and to achieve the best health outcome. Once I was looking after Ms Karma (pseudonym). She was a post- op day 1, cholecystectomy patient. In the clinical reasoning cycle, **first, I needed to consider the patient situation** and Ms karma's situation was post- op day 1 and the operation procedure was cholecystectomy. **The second step** is collect cues/ information. In this step, I observed that she was looking pale, unwell and stated to me that she was feeling weak. So, I gathered additional information by checking the wound location and signs of any infection. I checked the previous observation chart of the patient and found that her blood pressure was lower than the normal range. I did the set of observations, and her blood pressure was 82/59 mmHg, respiratory rate 16/ per minute, heart rate 95 bpm, oxygen saturation SPO2 97% and the temperature was 36.4.

I processed the information which was gathered and found that her wound site was normal and vital signs were within normal range. However, the blood pressure was lower than the normal range. The patient was hypotensive. **I identified the problems**

and issues by processing the information that blood loss in the surgery or inadequate fluid in the body can cause low blood pressure. I noticed that in her case if she had not got an immediate treatment, that could have caused hypovolemic shock.

I established the goal. I reported to my preceptor regarding her problem; he quickly confirmed my reading of blood pressure. The patient needed IV bolus fluids to increase fluid volume in the body immediately. **To take action, I contacted to the doctor immediately** to review the patient and the doctor came to the ward within 20 minutes and charted 1000mls fluid bolus IV infusion. **To evaluate the outcome**, after administering the fluid, I went and checked her vital signs, and her blood pressure was improved 100/70 mmhg. She was out of danger now, and she was saying to me that she was feeling better and her medical situations improved throughout the immediate action taken. In the clinical reasoning cycle, the last step is **reflecting on the process and new learning,** from that experience, I learnt to respond as quickly as possible and take immediate action to achieve safety and the best health outcome (Levett-Jones et al. 2009).

ISBAR (example Demonstration)

Thirdly, I used the **ISBAR** (Introduction, situation, background, assessment and recommendation) communication tool to communicate with the doctors effectively for the safety of the patient and to achieve the best health outcome. While contacting the doctor I clearly introduced myself for example by saying that I am Mohan Sangraula calling from level 8 south surgical ward. You need to mention the hospital name where you are working. I have a patient, Mr Joseph Malik (Pseudonym), 39-year-old gentleman. I am calling you at this time due to a high blood glucose level of Mr. Mallik. He is an insulin dependent diabetic patient and his blood glucose level is 13.5 mmol, (normal range of blood glucose level is

4-8 mmol). His vital signs are within normal range. I would like to recommend you review Mr. Mallik as soon as possible (This is ISBAR format of communication to the doctor to solve the problem of the patient, and this is an example demonstration only).

Critical Thinking and Analysis:

I always practiced with an evidence-based framework and participated in ongoing professional development (NMBA 2006). When I encountered new diseases and medicines, I researched in the reliable sources to understand its importance and implementation. Critical thinking and analysis are very important in nursing. This skill always helps you to find out the reason why you are doing this. For example, If the patient came to the hospital and he has the medication you can critically think about what sorts of medication the patient is having. All his medications might be related either to his medical history (related disease management) or to manage his presenting problem. There should be a direct relationship between the patient problems and the medication he is having. If you encounter any medicine inappropriately charted by the doctor your job is to remind the doctor about it and correct the mistake if it was made. If you are not 100% sure, you should not act on it. You need to clarify with the respective doctor or medical officer before you act. Ensure 100% patient safety at all times. Critical thinking is one of the fundamental tools of the nursing process (Maneval et al. 2011) which is defined as collecting, interpreting, analysing, synthesizing and evaluating care. It is more broadly defined as being able to draw upon knowledge as well as available information to formulate the conclusion of the problem (Maneval et al. 2011).

Critical thinking is actually considered the cognitive component for clinical reasoning and clinical judgment and is inherent in making sound clinical reasoning decisions (Maneval et al. 2011).

It means that you need to seek knowledge on how the particular patient can be managed. For that reason, you need to have an understanding of clinical guidelines, important diseases and how they are treated and managed in the ward. You can do research in the ward gathering information regarding the disease and treatment processes from the ward where you are working. Some of the important information I have gathered you can read to make a good understanding to help in your clinical placement and these things you may frequently encounter and these are as follows. For example, how do you provide nursing care management to post-op thyroid surgery patient?

Post op: Sitting up at least 45 degrees.

Analgesia for pain- You need to manage his pain. For that, you need to make sure the doctor has charted analgesia.

Monitor for swelling / Respiratory distress: Since oedema of the glottis or an injury to the recurrent laryngeal nerve can occur that can lead to a compromised airway (Sanderson & Allison 2007). In this situation, you need to observe the patient closely.

Drain Care: Because there is only a small amount of dead space in the neck, even a small amount of blood can cause airway obstruction. Drain output / redness needs to be closely monitored and documented. Wounds will normally be covered with steri-strips (do not place any large dressing over the site, as it will obscure the view) (Sanderson & Allison 2007).

Encourage mobility- You need to encourage his mobility so that the patient does not develop any clotting.

Calcium disturbance: The thyroid is the hormonal gland which produces thyroid hormone and calcitonin, whereas the parathyroid produces the parathyroid hormone. Calcitonin and parathyroid hormones participate in the control of calcium in the system. Therefore, there is always the risk of hypocalcaemia (Sanderson & Allison 2007).

Sign and symptoms of hypocalcaemia: Spasms or tingling in hands and feet and muscular twitching.

Calcium levels can drop quickly but can be replaced by IV and / or PO supplements. Therefore, always keep cannula in situ for post- op patient (Sanderson & Allison 2007).

In any field, three things are significant to achieve an excellent outcome. These are eyesight or eye (dristhi), concentration or focus (dhayan) and target (lackshya). Wherever you look at any object or things, your concentration and focus go towards it by following your eyes. Focus is necessary to achieve any target you set. So, three combinations should be matched to successfully complete any work in the human history, dristhi, dhayan and lackshya. So, to complete the clinical placement in a hospital setting without a fearful environment you should know how the nursing roles are functioning in the hospital environment. How the nursing staff are managing a patient and what you should do. If you know the whole system and how the patient is managed effectively, you do not have any fear and hesitation to go to the hospital to do the PEP. Rather, you go there motivated, encouraged and eager to learn the practical skill to be a competent RN in the near future. To understand the bigger picture and nursing management you need to understand the perioperative concepts and nursing management. If you master these concepts, these practically work in a hospital clinical environment. What assignment did you do in the university and the marks you scored does not, in fact, prove you are competent in a clinical environment. So, I am mentioning now in this chapter the most valuable lesson for nurses who are committed to becoming a competent registered nurse. In this concept, how the nurses' function and how they manage their patients effectively in the hospital environment.

Perioperative addresses nursing roles appropriate to the three phases of surgical experience. These are preoperative, intraoperative and post-operative.

Preoperative Nursing Management in Hospital setting

Before the day of surgery

The preoperative phase begins when the surgical intervention is made and ends when the patient is transferred to the operating room (Farrell 2005). Nursing activities begin before the day of surgery by interviewing the patient which include not only the physical assessment but also an emotional assessment, identification of known allergies, previous anaesthetic history and any genetic problems which might affect the surgical result (Farrell 2005). Nurses need to make sure necessary tests have been completed. The nurse needs to arrange appropriate consultative services and provide patient preparatory education regarding recovery from anaesthesia and post -operative care needs (Farrell 2005). 'Under normal circumstances, the nurse does not ask the patient to sign the form or witness the patient's signature' (Farrell 2005). It is the surgeon's responsibility to provide appropriate information to the patient. The patient should be informed regarding the benefits of surgery, possible risks, alternatives, complications, disfigurement, disability and removal of any body parts as well as expectation in early and late post- operative period (Farrell 2005).

Nurses need to assert that before the psychoactive premedication is administered consent should be signed because these types of drugs affect the patient's judgment and decision-making capacity

(Farrell 2005). The valid consent can be signed by a patient over 18 years of age who has the mental capacity to do so (Farrell 2005). In the case of an unconscious patient, disabled and mentally ill, responsible family member preferably next of kin can sign the consent form. For that, state regulation and agency policy must be followed (Farrell 2005).

A patent can refuse to go for the surgery; it is his legal right. However, such information should be documented and relayed to the surgeon so that other arrangements can be made (Farrell 2005). For instance, the surgery may be rescheduled, or additional information and support may be provided to the patient and the family (Farrell 2005).

On the day of Surgery

The nurse needs to review patient teaching, check the name band, identify the patient identity and verify the surgical site. Nurses need to make sure the patient has signed the valid consent form and an intravenous infusion is started (Farrell 2005). Before sending the patient to the operation theatre, the nurse needs to obtain the patient's health history, physical examination data and vital signs should be conducted and noted and baseline data needs to established and recorded appropriately in the charts for future comparisons (Meeker & Rothrock, cited in Farrell 2005, p.407).

After thorough history investigation and physical examination any abnormality indication found. In this situation, blood tests, x- rays and other diagnostic tests are prescribed (Aitkenhead et al., cited in Farrell 2005, p.407).

Some Factors that affect preoperatively

Fluid status and nutrition: optimum level of nutrition is a vital factor to promote healing and resisting infection and other types of surgical complications (Braunschweig, Gomez & Sheean, cited in Farrell 2005, p. 407). Assessment of nutritional status of the patient, identify information regarding obesity, undernutrition, malnutrition, weight loss, deficiencies in specific nutrients, the effects of medication on nutrients, abnormalities and specific problem of the patient (Quinn, cited in Farrell 2005, p. 407) are important to know prior to operation. Measurement of waist circumference and body mass index can identify nutritional needs of the patient (Department of aging, cited in Farrell 2005, p. 407). Any nutritional deficiency, for example malnutrition, must be corrected before the surgery so that sufficient protein is available for tissue repair (King et al., cited in Farrell 2005, p. 407). Some of the important nutrients needed for wound healing are protein, Kilojoules, water, vitamin c, thiamine, niacin, riboflavin folic acid, vitamin B 12, vitamin A, vitamin K, iron and zinc (Farrell 2005). Electrolyte imbalances, dehydration, and hypovolaemia can cause problems in the patient who has comorbid medical conditions or aged patients (Farrell 2005). Mild volume deficits may be treated during surgery. However, to promote best possible preoperative condition, correct nutritional needs and electrolytes deficit, additional time may be needed (Farrell 2005).

Patient's respiratory status: A patient who has respiratory diseases such as asthma or COPD needs to be assessed carefully for current threat to their pulmonary status. The medication used by the patient also needs to be assessed because that may affect recovery (King & Sametana, cited in Farrell 2005, p. 407). The goal for the potential surgical patient is optimal respiratory function. The patient needs the teaching of breathing exercises and use of incentive spirometer if indicated (Farrell 2005). If the patient has a respiratory infection, surgery will be postponed (Farrell 2005).

In general, patients who smoke are urged to stop 6-8 weeks before surgery (Australian and New Zealand college of Anaesthetists (ANZCA), cited in Farrell 2005, p. 407). However, many patients won't follow this. Patients who won't follow this need to be counselled to stop smoking at least 12 hours prior to surgery. Research suggests that this can help to reduce adverse effects associated with smoking, for example, increased airway reactivity, decreased mucociliary clearance, psychological changes in the cardiovascular and immune systems (Shannon-Cain, Webster & Cain, cited in Farrell 2005, p. 407).

Use of alcohol and drug: Acutely intoxicated persons are prone to injury. Therefore, surgery needs to postponed if it is possible. In the case of emergency, when surgery is required, local, spinal or reginal block anaesthesia is used for minor surgery patients (Farrell 2005). Otherwise, a nasogastric tube is inserted to prevent the patient from vomiting by aspirating the stomach contents before administering general anaesthesia (Farrell 2005). The person who has a history of chronic alcoholism often suffers from malnutrition and other types of systemic problems which may increase surgical risk (Farrell 2005).

Status of cardiovascular: In the preoperative period a well-functioning cardiovascular system is important to maintain oxygen, fluid and nutrition needs of the patient. If the patient has uncontrolled hypertension, surgery may be postponed until the blood pressure is controlled (Farrell 2005).

Renal and Hepatic function: The pre- operative goal is good function of the liver and the urinary system so that anaesthetic agents, medications, body wastes and toxins are adequately processed and remove from the body (Farrell 2005). The role of the liver is significant in the biotransformation of anaesthetic compounds. Thus, disorders in liver effects how anaesthetic agents are metabolised. For example, acute liver disease is associated with high surgical mortality so preoperatively improvement of liver function is the goal (Farrell 2005). Careful assessment of liver and various liver function tests may be required preoperatively (Farrell 2005).

Good function of the kidneys is important preoperatively because they are involved in excreting anaesthetic and their metabolites (Farrell 2005). While considering anaesthetic administration, it is important to know the acid-base status and metabolism (Farrell 2005). Surgery is contraindicated when the patient has acute nephritis, acute renal insufficiency with anuria, oliguria or acute renal problems (Farrell 2005).

Endocrine Function: When undergoing surgery, patients are at risk of hypoglycaemia and hyperglycaemia (Farrell 2005). Hypoglycaemia may develop during anaesthesia or postoperatively from inadequate carbohydrates or from excessive use of insulin (Farrell 2005). Hyperglycaemia may increase the risk of surgical wound infection (Farrell 2005). The goal is to maintain the blood glucose level between 3.5 and 5.5mmol (Farrell 2005). Frequent glucose monitoring is important before, during and after surgery (Farrell 2005).

Patients who has uncontrolled thyroid disorders are at risk of thyroid rotoxicosis (with hyperthyroid disorders) and respiratory failure (with hypothyroid disorders) (Farrell 2005). A patient who has received corticosteroids is at risk of adrenal insufficiency (Farrell 2005). Thus, use of corticosteroid must be reported to the surgeon and anaesthetist. Therefore, it is important to assess the patient for a history of these disorders (Farrell 2005).

The immune function: It is important to assess and document all the allergies and adverse drug reactions including medications, blood transfusion, contrast agents, latex and food products (Farrell 2005). Immunosuppression is common with chemotherapy, renal transplantation, radiation therapy and disorders affecting the immune system, for example, AIDS and leukaemia (Farrell 2005). The mildest symptoms or slightest temperature must be investigated because patients who are immunosuppressed are highly prone to infection (Farrell 2005).

Use of previous medication: Any medication the patient is using and has used in the past is documented including over the counter (OCT) preparations and herbal agents and the frequency which they are used (Farrell 2005). These medications might have interactions with anaesthetic agents that can cause a serious problem. For example, warfarin (Marevan) can increase the risk of bleeding during the intraoperative and post- operative period (Farrell 2005). Therefore, it should be discontinued in anticipation of elective surgery (Farrell 2005). The surgeon will determine how long before the elective surgery the patient should stop taking an anticoagulant, depending on the type of procedure and the medical condition of the patient (Farrell 2005).

Nursing intervention of immediate preoperative and patient preparation

The patient needs to wear a hospital gown, and the gown should be left untied and open in the back (Farrell 2005). The head needs to be covered with a disposable hair cap. The mouth needs to be inspected, and dentures should be removed but must remain with the patient (Farrell 2005). Any jewellery worn by the patient should be removed (Farrell 2005). All devices, for example, glasses and prosthetic devices are given to family members or labelled with the patient's name and stored in a safe place according to the hospital's policy (Farrell 2005).

All patients should void except those with urologic disorders before going to the operation theatre to promote continence during low abdominal surgery and to make abdominal organs more accessible. Urinary catheterization may be performed in the operation theatre as needed (Farrell 2005).

Filling the pre- operative checklist and maintaining record

Nurses need to fill up the preoperative checklist before sending the patient to the operation theatre. The completed chart accompanies the patient to the theatre with a surgical consent form attached along with all the laboratory reports and patient records (Farrell 2005). Any last-minute observations that may have a bearing on anaesthesia or surgery are noted at the front of the chart in a prominent place (Farrell 2005).

Patient transfer to the pre-surgical area

The patient will transfer to the operation suite in a bed or stretcher about 30 to 60 minutes before the anaesthetic is to be given (Farrell 2005). The stretcher or bed should be comfortable, and enough blankets need to be provided to prevent chilling in an air-conditioned room (Farrell 2005). A small head pillow is provided. The patient is taken to the anaesthetic bay, greeted by name, and positioned comfortably on the bed (Farrell 2005). The surrounding area should be quiet if the preoperative medication is to have maximum effect. Unpleasant sounds and conversations should be avoided because sedated patients may overhear and might misinterpret them (Farrell 2005).

Nursing management in intraoperative period

Surgical team

The surgical team involves the patient, anaesthetist, surgeons and their assistants. Throughout the surgery, an anaesthetist monitors the patient's physical status, and the main role is to administer the anaesthetic agent (Farrell 2005). The anaesthetic nurse assists the anaesthetist during induction, maintenance, and reversal of anaesthesia (Farrell 2005). The surgeon and assistant scrub perform the surgery. The scrub nurse provides sterile instruments and supplies to the surgeon during the operation procedure (Farrell 2005). The circulating nurse coordinates the care of the patient in the theatre (Farrell 2005). The care provided by the circulating nurse includes assisting the patient with positioning, preparation of the patient's skin for surgery, managing surgical specimens and documenting intraoperative events (Farrell 2005).

Nursing Care in the Intraoperative Period

During the surgery, nursing care management includes, providing for the safety and well- being of the patient, coordinating the operating room personnel, perform scrub and circulating activities (Farrell 2005). The care begins by the pre- operative nurse. For example, providing information and realistic reassurance is continued by the intraoperative nursing staff (Farrell 2005). The nurse supports the coping strategies and reinforces the patient's ability to influence outcomes by encouraging his or her active participation in the plan of care (Farrell 2005).

The intraoperative nurses' role is to advocate the patient and monitor factors that can cause injury, for example, patient position, equipment malfunction, and environmental hazards, and they protect patients' dignity and interests while they are anaesthetised

(Farrell 2005). In addition to that, they need to maintain the surgical standard of care, identifying existing risk factors, and assisting in modifying complicating factors to help reduce operative risk (Phippen & Wells, cited in Farrell 2005, p. 423).

Some potential Intraoperative complications

Nausea and vomiting is potential in the intraoperative period. If gagging occurs, the patient is turned to the side, the head of the table is lowered, and a basin is provided to collect the vomit (Farrell 2005). Suction is performed to remove saliva and vomited gastric contents (Farrell 2005). In some cases, the anaesthetist administers antimetics preoperatively or intraoperatively to counteract possible aspiration (Farrell 2005).

Anaphylaxis is caused due to medications reaction. Therefore, nurses need to be aware of the type and method of the anaesthesia and the specific agents used (Farrell 2005). An anaphylactic reaction can occur in response to many medications, latex or other substances. The reaction may be delayed or immediate (Farrell 2005). The anaphylaxis is a life-threatening acute allergic reaction which can cause bronchial constriction, vasodilation, and hypotension (Fortunato- Phillips, cited in Farrell 2005, p. 434). An anaphylactic shock may occur in patients already exposed to an antigen which have developed antibodies to it; it can often be prevented (Farrell 2005). To prevent an anaphylaxis, nurses need to assess all patients for allergies or previous reaction to antigens, for example, blood products, medications, foods, latex and contrast agents (Farrell 2005). When the new allergies are identified, the nurse needs to advise patients to wear or carry identification that names the specific allergies or antigen (Farrell 2005). The nurse must check or observe whether the patient is allergic to any medication prior to administering the medication (Farrell 2005).

Respiratory complications and Hypoxia: There are many potential problems with general anaesthesia, for example, inadequate ventilation, occlusion of the airway, inadvertent intubation of the oesophagus and hypoxia (Farrell 2005). The exchange of gases can lead to compromise due to respiratory depression caused by anaesthetic agents, aspiration of respiratory tract secretion or vomitus and the patient's position on the operating table (Farrell 2005). Hypoxia can cause brain damage within minutes. Therefore, vigilant assessment of the patient's oxygenation status is a primary function of the anaesthetist and the anaesthetist nurse (Farrell 2005). Peripheral perfusion is frequently checked, and pulse oximetry values need to be monitored continuously (Farrell 2005).

Hypothermia: In the period of anaesthesia, generally, the patient's temperature may fall. Glucose metabolism is reduced and due to that metabolic acidosis may develop (Farrell 2005). This condition is called hypothermia and is indicated by core body temperature below normal, 36 degrees C or lower (Farrell 2005). Hypothermia may occur because of a low temperature in the operation room, infusion of cold fluids, inhalation of cold gases, pharmacological agents, advanced age, open body wounds and cavity (Farrell 2005). Hypothermia may be intentionally induced, for example, cardiac surgery requiring a cardiopulmonary bypass to reduce the patient's metabolic rate (Finkelmeier, cited in Farrell 2005, p. 435).

If hypothermia occurs, the intervention is to minimise or reverse the physiologic process. If the hypothermia is intentional, the goal is to safely return normal body temperature (Farrell 2005). To prevent hypothermia, wet gowns and drapes should be removed promptly and replaced with dry materials because wet linen materials promote heat loss (Farrell 2005). Gradually, the patient must be rewarmed. Forced air warming blankets may be used.

Monitoring of core temperature, urinary output, arterial blood gas levels, ECG, blood pressure and serum electrolytes level is required (Farrell 2005).

Post anaesthetic recovery unit (PARU)

Post- anaesthetic care in a day surgical unit is divided into two phases (Farrell 2005). Phase 1 PARU is used to provide intensive care during the immediate recovery phase (Farrell 2005). The II phases of PARU are for the patient who requires less frequent observation and less nursing care (Farrell 2005). The patient may remain in a phase II PARU unit for as long as 4 to 6 hours, depending upon the type of surgery and any pre-existing conditions of the patient (Farrell 2005).

The nurse performs a baseline assessment, then checks the surgical site for drainage or haemorrhages and make sure that all drainage tubes and monitoring lines are connected and functioning (Farrell 2005).

In Phase I PARU, every 15 minutes, nurses provide monitoring of the patient's pulse, respiratory rate, electrocardiogram and pulse oximeter value (blood oxygen level) (Farrell 2005). In some cases, end -tidal carbon dioxide (ETCO) levels are monitored (Farrell 2005). Due to the effects of anaesthesia, a patient's airway may become obstructed, and the PARU nurse must be prepared to assist in reintubation and in handling other emergencies that may occur (Farrell 2005). The nurse in the phase II PARU must possess strong clinical assessment and patient teaching skill (Farrell 2005).

Frequent assessment of blood oxygen saturation level, depth and nature of respiration, pulse rate, and regularity, the level of consciousness, skin colour, and ability to respond to commands are the cornerstone of nursing care in PARU (Farrell 2005).

The patient remains in the PARU until they are fully recovered from anaesthetic agents (Hartfield & Tronson, cited in Farrell 2005, p. 445). Indicators of recovery include adequate respiratory function, stable blood pressure, adequate oxygen saturation level compared with baseline, spontaneous movement or movement on command, orientation to person, place, events and time, urine output at least 30 ml/h, nausea and vomiting absent or under control and minimal pain (Farrell 2005). These are the measures to determine the patient's readiness for discharge from the PARU (Farrell 2005).

Receiving the patient in ward

The first thing nurses need to do is make the bed available for a new patient by assembling the necessary equipment and supplies, for example, IV pole, emesis basin, drainage receptacle holder, tissues, disposable pads, blankets and post-operative charting forms (Farrell 2005). When the call is received from the PARU for patient transfer the additional patient items may be needed; that must be communicated (Farrell 2005). The PARU nurse gives the handover to the ward nurse, for example, the baseline data and the condition of the patient (Farrell 2005). The handover may include medical diagnosis, demographic data, procedure performed, allergies, comorbid conditions, unexpected intraoperative events, estimated blood loss, the type and amounts of fluid received, administration of pain medication, urine output, and information that the patient and family have received about the patient's condition. Generally, the surgeon speaks to the family member after the surgery (Farrell 2005).

The receiving nurse reviews the postoperative orders, admits the patient in the ward, performs an initial assessment, attends to the patient's immediate needs and prepares the care plan (Farrell 2005).

Post- operative care and Nursing management

Post- operative nursing care during the first 24 hours after surgery in a medical and surgical ward involves helping the patient recover from the effects of anaesthesia, assessing physiologic status of the patient, managing pain, monitoring for complications, implementing measures to achieve independence with self- care, successful management of the therapeutic regime, discharge to home and complete recovery (Farrell 2005).

Initial phase in the ward

In the initial hours when a patient is admitted to the ward, the primary concern and nursing care are the management of haemodynamic stability, adequate ventilation, surgical site integrity, incisional pain, nausea and vomiting, neurologic status and spontaneous voiding (Farrell 2005).

The pulse rate, respiration rate, and blood pressure are recorded at least every 15 minutes for the first hour and every 30 minutes for the next two hours (Farrell 2005). The temperature is monitored every four hours for the first 24 hours (Farrell 2005). Thereafter, they are measured less frequently if they remain stable for example, fourth hourly and sixth hourly per the requirement (Farrell 2005).

Several hours after surgery

Several hours after surgery or after waking up the next morning, the patient usually starts to feel better (Farrell 2005). Even though pain still is intense, many patients may feel more alert, less anxious and less nauseous (Farrell 2005). They start to breathe normally and commence leg exercise (Farrell 2005). Many of the patients may dangle their legs over the edge of the bed, stand and walk a few meters or assisted to sit on a chair (Farrell 2005). At this time, many patients will be able to tolerate a light diet and had IV fluid discontinued (Farrell 2005).

'The focus of care shifts from intense physiologic management and symptomatic relief of the adverse effects of anaesthesia to regaining independence with self- care and preparing for discharge' (Farrell 2005). Despite these improvements, there are still some risks of complication for a post- operative patient. These are as follows: pneumonia, atelectasis, deep vein thrombosis, constipation, pulmonary embolism, paralytic ileus and wound infection are ongoing threats for the post-operative patient (Farrell 2005).

What might Impact of surgery to the patient?

The body's fluid balance after surgery is determined by day to day net increase and loss of two components: water and its dominant electrolyte, sodium (Kayilioglu et al. 2015). Surgery can result in water, sodium, and potassium to move abnormally between fluid compartments (SVPH 2014). The permeability causes the movement of water, electrolytes and other particles into the interstitial space to allow the necessary factors to reach the site of the injury (SVPH 2014). The third space fluid shift leads to localised swelling and lymphatic blockage, causing localised interstitial oedema (SVPH 2014). This can result in the patient being 'dry' or hypovolemic, having a low circulating blood volume, as fluid has moved into the interstitial spaces (SVPH 2014).

The drugs administered during anaesthesia directly depress baroreceptor, renal and cardiac function, blunting the body's normal compensatory responses (Farrell 2005). You are likely to see low blood pressure and slow, less effective heartbeats. These effects can last for up to 24 hours following surgery (SVPH 2014).

In the first 12 to 48 hours following abdominal surgery, patients are in a dry or loss stage, when the intravascular spaces are depleted (SVPH 2014).

In this stage, patients might have hypertensive and hypotensive, dry mucous membranes, weight gain, oedema, elevated serum glucose, pale in skin, hypokalaemia, cool and atrial arrhythmias (SVPH 2014).

Sign and symptoms of fluid imbalance

Assessing fluid imbalance

Blood pressure
pulse
oedema and skin turgor
weight changes (Shephard 2011).
respiratory status
blood tests
urine output (SVPH 2014).

Blood pressure

Elevated blood pressure can indicate fluid overload. Elevated blood pressure also can indicate post-operative pain and anxiety

(Farrell 2005). Thus, other sign and symptoms also need to take consideration. For a lower blood pressure, there might be a 15-25% intravascular fluid deficit before systolic BP falls (Farrell 2005).

Pulse

Tachycardia can be a sign and symptom of either fluid deficit or overload. Another sign might be the stress to increase heart rate (Shephard 2011). To understand the patient's fluid imbalance, other signs also need to be taken into consideration (Shephard 2011).

Oedema and skin turgor

Unless patients are weighed daily, it's difficult to observe oedema. Patients who are on bed rest will show sacral swelling (SVPH 2014). Patients who are ambulatory will show swelling in their ankles, wrists and fingers. A decreased skin turgor can be a sign of fluid deficit (SVPH 2014).

Weight changes

1 litre of water is approximately equal to 1 kilogram. Any weight gain can be a sign of fluid overload (SVPH 2014). Patients who are in nil by mouth and having intravenous fluid can lose 0.3-0.5 kg a day (SVPH 2014). This should not be mistaken for dehydration (SVPH 2014).

Respiratory status

Fluid overload and pleural effusions can be assessed through lung sounds. The patient who has fluid overload or plural effusions might also have a decreased oxygen saturation level and dyspnoea (Farrell 2005).

Blood tests

A low haematocrit (HCT) can result from a dilution of the blood as fluid overload. An elevated HCT can point to fluid deficit (SVPH 2014). HCT can be low if the patient has bleeding (SVPH 2014). Reviewing the trend of a repeated HCT may be more useful. If the water is lost, then serum sodium will be elevated. If only water is gained, then sodium levels will be low (Farrell 2005).

What is the nursing management?

The best nursing management of fluid and electrolyte imbalance is prevention.

- You need to record intake and output which help to determine whether a positive or negative balance is being achieved (SVPH 2014).
- Make a record of the pulse (important if there is a potassium imbalance) and blood pressure (SVPH 2014).
- Maintain fluid replacement regimes, (either enternal or parenteral) at the correct rate (SVPH 2014).
- Observe the patient's skin (If the person is dehydrated their skin becomes inelastic) (SVPH 2014).
- Observe the patient's tongue and mucus membranes for dryness, and observe whether the degree of dryness makes speaking difficult (SVPH 2014).
- Observe the urine output (the urine of someone dehydrated is concentrated; the urine of someone overhydrated by contrast is dilute) (SVPH 2014).
- Observe the patient's mental state, disorientation and consciousness (SVPH 2014).

Post- operative dressing change

The first post-operative dressing is usually changed by a member of a surgical team. The other subsequent post -operative dressings are usually performed by the nurse. The dressing is applied to a wound for one or more of the following reasons (Farrell 2005).

- To provide an appropriate environment for wound healing (Farrell 2005).
- To absorb drainage (Farrell 2005).
- To immobilise the wound or splint (Farrell 2005).
- To protect the wound and new epithelial tissue from mechanical injury (Farrell 2005).
- To protect the wound from bacterial contamination and from soiling by faeces, urine, and vomitus (Farrell 2005).
- To promote haemostasis, as in a pressure dressing (Farrell 2005).
- To provide mental and physical comfort for the patient (Farrell 2005).

The nurse needs to tell the patient that changing the dressing is a simple procedure associated with little discomfort. Usually, dressing change is performed at a suitable time (for example, not at meal time or when a visitor is present) (Farrell 2005). Draw a curtain for privacy. Assurance needs to be given to the patient that the incision will shrink as it heals and the redness will fade (Farrell 2005). The nurse needs to perform hand hygiene before and after the dressing change and wear the disposable gloves to change the dressing (Farrell 2005). The tape or adhesive portion of the dressing is removed by pulling it parallel with the skin surface and in the direction of hair growth, rather than at right angles. Use of alcohol wipes or non-irritating solvents aid in removing adhesive painlessly and quickly (Farrell 2005). The old dressing is removed and then deposited in a container designated for biomedical waste disposal (Farrell 2005). Standard precaution should be performed, and the dressing should not be touched by ungloved hands because of risk involving transmission of pathogenic organism (Farrell 2005).

While changing the dressing, the nurse has an opportunity to teach the patient how to care for the incision and change the dressing at home as required (Farrell 2005).

Some possible drugs and supplements for post- op patient

Most of the post- op patient doctor's orders were antibiotics, antifungal, analgesics, antiemetic, IV fluids, anticoagulants, antacids or proton pump inhibitor.

Antibiotics

Antibiotics are being used to combat bacteria which cause infection (Munckhof 2005). IV antibiotics are most commonly given to the patient if they have any infection risk. Antibiotics can be given orally as well. Before administrating IV antibiotics, you always need to ask the patient if there is any history of antibiotic allergy to avoid the risk of reaction (Munckhof 2005). Most common antibiotics I used in the ward were third generation cephalosporins, for example, ceftriaxone.

Surgical antibiotics prophylaxis is given to the patient to prevent infections at the surgical sites. Appropriate surgical prophylaxis can decrease the risk of postoperative wound infections (Munckhof 2005). Commonly used surgical prophylactic antibiotics were as follows.

Intravenous (IV) 'first generation' cephalosporins - Cephalothin or cephazolin

IV gentamicin

IV metronidazole (Flagyl) - antifungal, if anaerobic infection is likely.

IV flucloxacillin (if methicillin - susceptible staphylococcal infection is likely).

IV vancomycin (if methicillin - susceptible staphylococcal infection is likely) (Munckhof 2005).

Post-operative analgesics

Patient- controlled analgesia (PCA) allows the patient to control the administration of their own medication within predetermined safety limits. Patients who use PCA achieve better pain relief. The main goal of the PCA is to achieve a minimum therapeutic level of analgesia and to allow the patient to maintain that level by using the PCA pumps (Farrell & Dempsey 2011).

Analgesia

For severe pain 7-10/10, a strong opioid for moderate to severe pain; for example, morphine.

For moderate pain 4-6/10, a weak opioid for mild to moderate pain; for example, codeine.

For mild pain 1-3/10, non -opioid; for example, aspirin, paracetamol or nonsteroidal anti-inflammatory drugs (NSAID) (World Health Organization 2015).

Deep vein thrombosis (DVT) prophylaxis

Deep vein thrombosis means a blood clot forms in a vein particularly in the leg (Cayley 2007). DVT is more common after surgery because the patient does not mobilise like normal. It can be prevented and treated by giving anticoagulants drugs that thin the blood and reduce the chance of clotting (Cayley 2007). DVT can create a serious problem if it begins to travel through the veins of the body. When a clot reaches the heart, it can be pumped through the bloodstream to the lungs, where a life-threatening pulmonary embolism can occur or can cause a stroke (Cayley 2007). To prevent clotting after surgery, the doctor prescribes anticoagulants drugs for example subcut heparin or enoxaparin. Graduated compression stockings and calf compressors also can reduce clot formation (Cayley 2007).

Intravenous (IV) fluids

Iv fluids are given to patients for mainly two reasons, for example, to replace fluids which they have lost through illness or injury. Another reason is to provide fluids when they are unable to drink. The fluids are selected based on the patients' need and can change periodically during hospital stay (National Institute for Health and Care Excellence (NIHCE) 2013). The common IV fluids are .45 NaCl (half normal saline,9 NaCl (normal saline) and 5% Dextrose (D5). 0.9% NaCl normal saline is isotonic, without glucose and use for initial volume resuscitation, for example, trauma and septic shock. Hartmann's solution is also isotonic without glucose which is often used intra- operatively and post-operatively (NIHCE 2013).

Electrolytes

Electrolytes are important compounds in the blood which can conduct an electrical charge and facilitate the body's complete essential functions, including helping the beating of the heart (Blann 2014). Too few electrolytes and too many electrolytes can bring disruptions in the heart and heart function or cause other serious problems (Blann 2014). For prevention of complications from electrolytes imbalances, supplements can be given orally or via IV. Electrolytes supplements are phosphorous (Potassium Phosphate), Calcium Chloride, Magnesium Chloride and Potassium Chloride (Blann 2014).

The major electrolytes are as follows

Sodium (NA+)
Potassium (K +)
Chloride (CL⁻)
Magnesium (Mg2+)
Bicarbonate (HCO3⁻)
Phosphate (PO42⁻)
Calcium (Ca2+)
Sulphate (SO42-) (Saladin 2012).

Antacids

Antacids are a common part of recovery from surgery. Even if patients are not well enough to eat or drink, their stomach continuous to produce stomach acids (Maton & Burton 1999). Antacids are given for gastric ulcers, stress gastritis and gastro-oesophageal reflux disease (GORD), for example Pantoprazole. Pantoprazole works by inhibiting the action of the proton pumps that reduces the production of stomach acid (Maton & Burton 1999).

Drain management

The most common drains in the ward are Redivac and Jackson - Pratt (JP) drains. The drains will drain excess fluids from the operation site. Over a few days the colour changes from thick frank blood to haemoserous to serous (Walker 2007). Drains are emptied every 24hrs at 2400hrs usually at midnight. Drains are to be secured and checked for no kinks/ clamps are set correctly (Walker 2007).

Stoma observation

The size and the shape of the stoma changes significantly from immediately post-op to the time of discharge. Observations should take place for at least 48hrs post-op and be documented on a stoma observation chart (Burch 2013).

Observation includes: Colour (pink, red dusky, black).
: Temperature (warm, cool, cold)
: Output (Nil, serous, haemoserous, green, brown) (Burch 2013).

Output: The amount of output needs to be measured and documented on the fluid balance chart. Ileostomy output can be quite watery and high when newly formed. Therefore, the patient may need IV fluids to keep hydrated during this stage (Burch 2013).

Stoma education

Ostomy patients need to learn A) how to empty the bag, B) how to change the bag, C) dietary changes, and D) activity changes by the time of discharge and provide them emotional support (Burch 2013).

You always need to use evidence-based practice resources to look after the patient under your care. You need to use critical thinking and analysis to reflect yourself by asking a question such as what are you doing? and why are you doing it?

Pressure Ulcer Management in acute care nursing

Background (What are Pressure Ulcers?)

Pressure ulcer occurs when soft tissue is compressed between an external surface and a bony prominence for a long period of time (European Pressure Ulcer Advisory Panel and National Pressure Ulcer Advisory Panel (EPUAP & NPUAP) 2009).

Factors contribute to pressure ulcers

Pressure Ulcer

Impaired mobility, impaired activity, impaired sensory function (Woodward 1999).

Extrinsic factors

Moisture, shear, friction (Woodward 1999).

Intrinsic factors

Poor nutrition, poor oxygen delivery, skin temperature and chronic illness (Woodward 1999).

Common pressure ulcers sites

Supine: 23% sacro-coccygeal, 8% heels, 1% Occiuput; spine (Myers 2004).

Sitting:

24% ischium
3% elbows (Myers 2004).

Lateral:

15% trochanter
7% malleolus
6% knee
3% heels (Myers 2004).

Rational behind developing pressure ulcer

A pressure ulcer can develop within two weeks of hospital admission. The elderly can develop pressure ulcers within the first week of admission. Initial assessment is required upon admission and repeated at least 24-48 hours (EPUAP & NPUAP 2009).

Assessment (Waterlow)

Developed in 1985, gives an estimated risk for the development of pressure sore in a given patient.

Scoring criteria

Body mass index (BMI) including weight and height, skin type, sex and age, malnutrition screening tool, continence, mobility, tissue malnutrition, Neurological deficit and major surgery or trauma (as an additional checklist).

Waterlow score >10 indicates risk of pressure ulcer, >15 high risk and greater than 20 very high risk developing pressure ulcer (National Safety and Quality Health Service (NSQHS) 2012).

Classification of pressure ulcer

Stages I, II, III, IV, suspected deep tissue injury (DTI), unstageable. The staging of pressure ulcer reflects the amount of tissue damage (EPUAP & NPUAP 2009).

Rational behind dressing change and applying hydrogel

Daily dressing change can prevent the infection. Hydrogel is a water-based gel which is called amorphous that can re- hydrate dry slough and necrotic tissue to create moist and wound healing environment (Purser 2009).

Stage I pressure ulcer

'Intact skin with non -blanchable erythemia of a localized area usually over a bony prominence' (EPUAP & NPUAP 2009, p.30).

Nursing intervention

Keep area clean and dry, incontinence management

Use moisture barrier cream PRN, turning and repositioning schedule.

Stage II Pressure Ulcer

'Partial thickness loss of dermis with a red, pink wound bed without slough' (EPUAP & NPUAP) 2009, p.30).

Intervention

Use normal saline to clean the wound. Apply a small amount of hydrogel and use non-adherent dressing to cover the wound and change the dressing every day (Myers 2004).

Turning and repositioning schedule and off the load area of the pressure ulcer with pressure reducing (Myers 2004).

Stage III pressure Ulcer

'Full thickness tissue loss. Subcutaneous fat may be visible but bone, tendon or muscles are not exposed, and slough may be present' (EPUAP & NPUAP) 2009, p.30).

Intervention

Use normal saline to clean the wound. Apply a small amount of hydrogel and use non-adherent dressing to cover the wound and change the dressing every day (Myers 2004).

Turning and repositioning schedule and off the load area of the pressure ulcer with pressure reducing (Myers 2004).

Presence of slough with drainage

Use calcium alginate or foam dressing for moderate to copious drainage management (Myers 2004).

Negative pressure wound therapy is preferred treatment if slough in the wound 30 % or less (Myers 2004).

Stage IV Pressure Ulcer

With exposed bone, full thickness tissue loss tendon or muscle (EPUAP & NPUAP 2009).

Intervention

Use normal saline to clean the wound. Apply a small amount of hydrogel and use non-adherent dressing to cover the wound and change the dressing every day (Myers 2004).

Off load area of the pressure ulcer with a pressure relieving, turning and repositioning schedule.

Presence of slough with drainage

Use calcium alginate or foam dressing for moderate to copious drainage management.

Negative pressure wound therapy is preferred treatment if slough 30% or less in the wound.

Tunnelling and undermining shall be filled appropriately.

Prevention is the key intervention for pressure ulcer injury

Provide good nutrition to the patient, **repositioning every two hourly**. Avoid skin friction and shear forces, use transfer aids to reduce friction and shear forces, air mattress, cushion, sheepskin, skin inspection regularly, checking the tubing site and **attending the pressure area.** Care, assessment and documentation are required (EPUAP & NPUAP 2009).

Blood Pressure

Blood pressure is the force that the blood exerts against a vessel wall (Saladin 2012). It can be measured within a blood vessel or the heart by inserting a catheter or needle connected to an external manometer (pressure measuring device) (Saladin 2012). It is measured by a sphygmomanometer connected to an inflatable cuff wrapped around the arm. The brachial artery passing through this region is close to the heart that the BP recorded here approximates the maximum arterial BP found anywhere in the body (Saladin 2012).

Systolic Pressure

Systolic pressure is the peak arterial BP attending during ventricular contraction (Saladin 2012). According to Vaughn's blood pressure chart, systolic 70-90 low blood pressure (hypotension), 90-120 ideal blood pressure, 120-140 pre- high blood pressure, 140-190 high blood pressure (hypertension).

Diastolic pressure

Diastolic pressure is the minimum arterial BP occurring during the ventricular relaxation between heartbeats (Saladin 2012).

According to Vaughn's blood pressure chart, diastolic pressure 40-60 low blood pressure (hypotension), 60-80 ideal blood pressure, 80-90 pre- high blood pressure and 90-100 high blood pressure (hypertension).

Before giving cardiac medications, you need to check the patient's blood pressure. You should not give these tablets if the patient's blood pressure is low. If you gave it to the patient, it can cause more problems for the patient. So, you should not give cardiac meds during this condition. You need to ask the doctor to review the medication. You need to mention the reason you did not give it to the patient in your progress notes, and make sure you handed it to next shift RN. The preceptor and facilitator would like to observe how you respond in the clinical situation and whether you practice safely or not. So, always remember to check the blood pressure (BP) of the patient before giving cardiac medication. So, you need to have an understanding of what sorts of cardiac medication patient might have. I will explain some of them and please study before going to the PEP.

1. Angiotensin- converting enzymes (ACE) inhibitors

Mechanism of action: Prevent angiotensin – converting enzyme (ACE) that is used in the conversion of angiotensin I to II. Angiotensin II, in fact, stimulates the synthesis and secretion of aldosterone which causes raising blood pressure via a potent vasoconstrictor effect (CCU 2014).

Indication: Hypertension, heart failure, post MI

Common adverse reactions: Hypotension, persistent dry cough, renal impairment, hyperkalaemia (CCU 2014).

Medicine examples: Captopril, Enalapril, Ramipril, Lisinopril, Perindopril, Quinapril

Easy to remember because all have a common suffix, pril.

2. Angiotensin II receptor antagonist

Mechanism of action and /indications are similar to ACE inhibitors., but the difference is less likely to have a persistent dry cough (CCU 2014).

Medication examples: Candesartan, Losartan, Telmisartan

3. Beta – Blockers

Mechanism of action: This medication acts on beta 1 receptors which are found mostly in the heart, and it reduces heart rate and force of constriction (CCU 2014). And on beta -2 receptors, found mostly in bronchial and vascular smooth muscle cells. Therefore, may cause bronchial and vasoconstriction (CCU 2014).

Indications: Ischaemic heart disease, hypertension, arrhythmias, cardiac failure—but not in the acute phase (CCU 2014).

Adverse effects: Hypotension, bardycardia/ heart block, prolonged QT interval (Sotalol), bronchospasm, lethargy, erectile dysfunction (CCU 2014).

Examples medications: Metoprolol, Carvedilol, Sotalol, Bisoprolol

4. Calcium Channel blockers

Mechanism of action: Prevent entry of calcium into cells, causing vasodilation and smooth muscle relaxation, therefore, reducing blood pressure (CCU 2014). Some calcium channel blockers prolong AV node conduction time and reduce SA node conduction, and this may cause reducing heart rate (CCU 2014).

Indication: Angina, hypertension, arrhythmias (CCU 2014).

Adverse effects: Hypotension, bradycardia, worsening cardiac failure, headache/ flushing (CCU 2014).

Medication examples: Diltiazem, Verapamil, Nifedipine, Amolodipine, Felodipine (CCU 2014).

5. Diuretics

Loop diuretics: produce intense diuresis of relatively short duration, for example Frusemide, which prevents sodium and chloride absorption in the ascending loop of Henley and both proximal and distal tubules (CCU 2014).

Potassium -sparing diuretics – relatively weak diuretic and normally used in conjunction with loop diuretic of thiazide for example spironolactone. It may be used to treat persistent hypokalaemia (CCU 2014).

Thiazides: Prevent sodium and chloride reabsorption in the kidney tubules producing an increase in potassium excretion, for example, bendrofluazide, indipamide, hydrochlorothiazide (CCU 2014).

Indications: Hypertension, congestive cardiac failure

Adverse effects: Electrolyte depletion, dehydration and possible renal failure, hyperkalaemia, hyperuricaemia, hyperglycaemia, hypercholesterolemia (CCU 2014).

6. Statins

Mechanism of action: Prevents synthesis of cholesterol in liver

Indications: Hypercholesterolemia

Adverse effects: GI irritation, hepatic impairment, headache, nightmares

Consideration

Given at night as most cholesterol synthesis occurs at this time (CCU 2014).

Can interact with other medications, for example, increases blood concentration level of warfarin, digoxin, erythromycin (CCU 2014).

7. Nitrates

Mechanism of action: cause coronary artery and systemic vasodilation, therefore, decreasing the oxygen requirements of the myocardium and reducing blood pressure. Pre- load and cardiac workload is reduced (CCU 2014).

Indications: ischaemic heart disease, congestive cardiac failure, pulmonary hypertension (CCU 2014).

Adverse effects: Hypotension, tachycardia, headache, flushing

Medications examples:

Sublingual GTN (Anginine)

GTN patch (must be removed to allow patients 8 hours free of nitrates to prevent tolerance)

IV GTN must be administered in a glass bottle and non- PVC infusion set as GTN is absorbed by plastic.

Isosorbide mononitrate (IMDUR) long-acting tablets (CCU 2014).

Some important pharmacology

1) Mr Campbell has complained of chest pain. He is ordered Anginine. How is this medication administered and what are your nursing responsibilities post administration?

Answer:

Sublingually
Assess chest pain of the patient: for example, is it relieved or not?
Assess blood pressure
Assess adverse reactions, for example: headache (Tiziani 2010)

2) For mild analgesia, paracetamol is often used in the acute care setting. What is the main complication of overdose paracetamol?

Hepatic necrosis (Tiziani 2010).

3) Metformin is mostly used for type 2 diabetes patients. What is the action of Metformin?

Increases insulin sensitivity thought to prevent gluconeogenesis in the liver and glucose absorption from the gastrointestinal tract (Tiziani 2010).

4) Patient's ordered is IM morphine. What is the purpose of this medication and what is the process of administration of a schedule 8 medication?

It is a strong analgesia (Tiziani 2010).
Locked cupboard
2 RNs to check and sign
Same 2 RNs at the bedside for checks
Must be 2 RNs present until medication is given

2 signatures in DD book

5) What class of drug is aspirin and how does it work?

It is an antiplatelet. Antiplatelet agents inhibit unwanted thrombus formation by decreasing platelet aggregation (Tiziani 2010).

6) Prior to attending the operating suite for an ORIF the attending medical officer prescribed Miss Catherine a stat dose 1-gram Ceftriaxone to be given IV (intravenous) at 1600

Why this medication ordered for the patient?

Prophylactic antibiotic, broad spectrum (Tiziani 2010).

7) You are to administer as a push dose. Please list 4 nursing considerations not including the five rights.

IV cannula site: patent, not red or sore
Size of cannula
Check what diluent to use water or the normal saline in Australian injectable drug guide book online through CIAP or book
Slow administration 3-5 minutes
Have they had the medication before? May be allergic and does not know compatibility with IV solution running if they have some.

8) What type of drug is atorvastatin and how does it work?

Statin (HMG-CoA reductase inhibitor)
Reduce cholesterol significantly in patients with type II hyperlipidaemia (Tiziani 2010).

9) You are to administer Enaxaparin S/C, please list four nursing consideration when administering this medication?

Site rotation
Skin integrity observation
Any sign and symptoms of bleeding or increasing bruising
Expiry date
Do not rub the site after injection (Tiziani 2010).

10) You are administering Act rapid to a client, list four nursing consideration when administering this medication?

Blood glucose level
Time of the blood sample check
Is the patient able to eat?
Site rotation
Angle of needle 45 or 90 depending on amount of subcutaneous fat the client has
Skin integrity at the site of injection (Tiziani 2010).

11) What is the action of GTN?

Potent vasodilator: relaxes smooth muscle including vascular muscle causing relaxation
vasodilation (Tiziani 2010).

What assessment is done prior to administering GTN?

Blood pressure (Tiziani 2010).

12) What assessments should be made following administration of GTN?

Blood pressure
Chest pain assessment
Assess for any adverse effects (Tiziani 2010).

Diabetics are very common, and you will encounter these patients in most of the wards.

Managing type 1 diabetes

In type 1 diabetes, the pancreas produces insufficient or absence of insulin which is significant for converting glucose into energy. Therefore, people with diabetes needs to do the job of the pancreas by replacing the insulin via insulin injection or an insulin pump (Diabetes Australia (DA) 2015). The insulin reduces the level of glucose in the blood. Type 1 diabetes is a life-threatening condition that needs to be closely managed. The following are the strategies to manage type 1 diabetes (Diabetes Australia (DA) 2015).

- insulin replacement through lifelong insulin injections or use of an insulin pump
- monitored of blood glucose levels regularly as directed by a doctor
- strictly by following healthy diet and eating plan
- doing regular exercises

To manage type 1 diabetes, blood glucose level as close to the target range as possible between 4 to 6 mmol/l (fasting) (Diabetes Australia (DA) 2015).

Managing Type 2 diabetes

In type 2 diabetes, the pancreas is still working but not as effectively as it needs to. This means that the body is building insulin resistance and is unable to effectively convert glucose into energy leaving too much glucose in the blood (DA 2015). Type 2 diabetes can initially be managed through modification of lifestyle including exercise, healthy diet and monitoring your blood glucose levels (DA 2015). Type 2 diabetes is a progressive condition. As time progresses, the insulin becomes more resistant, and the pancreas becomes less effective converting glucose into energy (DA 2015). To help the pancreas convert glucose into energy, people with type 2 diabetes are often prescribed tablets to control their blood glucose levels (DA 2015). The objective of diabetes management is to keep blood glucose levels as close to the target range 4 to 6 mmol/l (fasting). This will help prevent both short-term and long-term complications (DA 2015). The tablets or injections are intended to be used together with healthy eating and regular physical activity (Diabetes Australia (DA) 2015).

Hypoglycaemia

Hypoglycaemia is a condition that happens when a person's blood glucose level has dropped too low, below 4mmol/l (DA 2015). It is significant to treat a hypo quickly to stop the BGL from falling even lower, and the person becomes seriously unwell (Diabetes Australia (DA) 2015).

Hypoglycaemia only occurs in people who take insulin or certain glucose-lowering tablets. People who manage their diabetes with healthy eating and physical activity are not at risk of hypo (Diabetes Australia (DA) 2015).

What may cause hypoglycaemia?

- excessive insulin or other glucose-lowering tablets
- missing a meal or delaying
- intake of fewer carbohydrates
- more strenuous exercise than usual
- drinking alcohol, more alcohol consumption can cause hypo (DA 2015).

Symptoms:

Early sign and symptoms may include the following

Dizziness, sweating, headache, hunger, paleness, shaking, trembling or weakness, pins and needles around mouth and mood change (DA 2015).

More serious symptoms include confusion, slurred speech, not able to drink or swallow, loss of consciousness, fitting /seizures (Diabetes Australia (DA) 2015).

Treating hypoglycaemia

Step 1.

- If the BGL is below 4mmol/l
- 6-7 jellybeans or
- 1/2 can of regular soft drink or
- 1/2 glass of fruit juice or
- 3 teaspoons of sugar or honey (Diabetes Australia (DA) 2015).

Step 2.

- Wait for 15 minutes and recheck the BGL to see if the BGL has increased above 4 mmol/l
- If the BGL is still below 4 mmol/l, repeat step 1 (DA 2015).

Step 3.

- Eat a snack or meal with longer acting carbohydrate for example:
- a slice of bread or

- a glass of milk or
- 1 piece of fruit or
- 2-3 pieces of dried apricots or
- pasta or rice (Diabetes Australia (DA) 2015).

What happens if not treated hypoglycaemia?

If hypoglycaemia not treated quickly, the BGL will continue to drop; that may result in the brain not getting enough glucose. This can cause unconsciousness or fitting (Diabetes Australia (DA) 2015).

What to do if the person is unconscious, drowsy or unable to swallow. It is a medical emergency. You need to clear the patient's airway by putting him on the side (DA 2015). For this situation, glucagon injection can be administered. Phone for the ambulance dial 000 stating that the person has diabetes (Diabetes Australia (DA) 2015).

What is glucagon?

Glucagon is a hormone that raises the BGL. It is injected into a muscle to reverse severe hypoglycaemia in people with diabetes (Diabetes Australia (DA) 2015).

Hyperglycaemic

Hyperglycaemia means high blood sugar level

Symptoms

- feeling excessive thirsty (DA 2015).
- frequently passing large volumes of urine
- feeling tired
- blurred vision (DA 2015).

- weight loss
- infections (e.g. thrush, cystitis, wound infections) (DA 2015).

Common causes

Sickness, infection, stress, consumption of too many carbohydrates, not enough insulin or diabetes tablets, other tablets or medicines (DA 2015).

Treatment

Contact a doctor if the patient has hyperglycaemic. If the patient has type 1 diabetes the doctor may prescribe insulin injection (DA 2015). If the patient has type 2 diabetes, the doctor may prescribe tablets to lower the BGL in normal range between 4-8 mmol /l (Diabetes Australia (DA) 2015).

Injection Administration

Intramuscular Injection

When other types of drug administered methods are not recommending for example oral, intravenous and subcutaneous, at this type of situation, intramuscular injection are used to administer the drug (Cafasso 2015). Intramuscular injection may be used instead of oral drug administration. With oral delivery, some drugs are destroyed by the digestive system after the drug is swallowed (Cafasso 2015). It may also be used instead of intravenous injection because some drugs are irritating to veins or if a suitable vein is not found (Cafasso 2015).

Intramuscular injection is absorbed faster than subcutaneous injection because muscle tissue has a larger blood supply than the tissue just under the skin for example subcutaneous tissue (Cafasso 2015). Muscle tissue also can hold a larger volume of the medication than the subcutaneous tissue (Cafasso 2015).

Deltoid muscle of the arm

Deltoid muscle injection site is typically used for vaccines and typically no more than 1ml because of its small muscle mass limits the volume of medication that can be injected (Cafasso 2015). For the exact location of this site to inject the medication, first feel for the bone that is called acromion process which is located at the top of the upper arm (Cafasso 2015). The correct site to give the injection is two finger widths below the acromion process (Cafasso 2015). At the bottom of the two fingers, there is an upside-down triangle. You can give the injection in the centre of the triangle; this is the correct location, to give injection on the Deltoid muscle (Cafasso 2015).

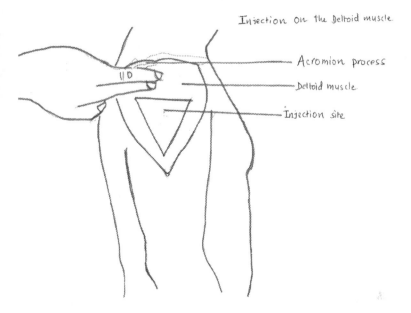

Injection on the Deltoid muscle

— Acromion process

— Deltoid muscle

— Injection site

(http://www.healthline.com)

Vastus Lateralis muscle of the thigh

The thigh may be used when the other site is not available. You need to divide the upper thigh into three equal parts. Locate the middle of these tree sections. The injection should go into the outer portion of this site (Cafasso 2015).

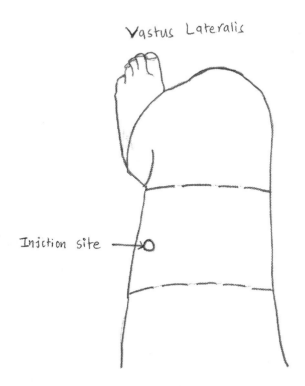

Vastus Lateralis

Injction site

(http://www.healthline.com)

Ventrogluteal muscle of the hip

This muscle is the safest site for adults and children older than seven months. It's deep and not close to any major blood vessels or nerves (Cafasso 2015).

You need to place the heel of your hand on the hip of the person receiving the injection, with the fingers pointing towards their head. Position the fingers so the thumb points towards the groin and you feel the pelvis under your pinkie finger (Cafasso 2015). You need to spread your index fingers in a slight "V" shape and inject the needle into the middle of that "V" (Cafasso 2015).

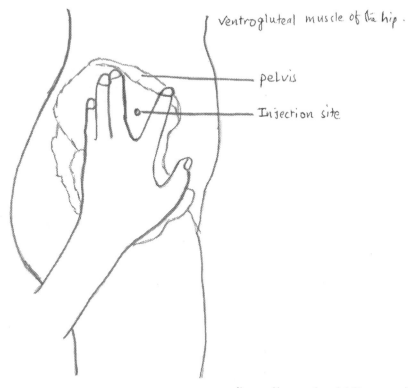

Ventrogluteal muscle of the hip.

pelvis

Injection site

(http://www.healthline.com)

Dorsogluteal muscles of the buttocks

The most commonly selected site for IM injection by healthcare providers is the dorsogluteal muscle of the buttocks (Cafasso 2015). You need to divide the buttock into four equal quadrants, halfway down from top to bottom and halfway across (Cafasso 2015). The IM injection should always go into the upper, outer quadrant of the buttock, towards the hip bone (Cafasso 2015).

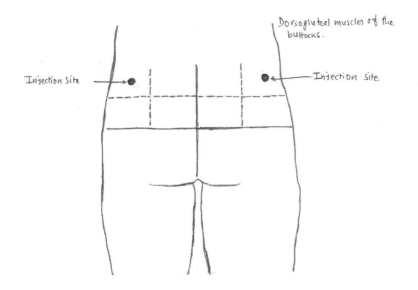

(http://www.healthline.com)

IM Injection procedure

- Wash your hands or hand hygiene
- Gather all needed supplies, for example, needle and syringe with medication, alcohol wipes, gauze, and a sharps container (Cafasso 2015).

Prepare syringe with medication

- Remove the cap of the vial, and the rubber stopper should be cleaned with an alcohol swab (Cafasso 2015).
- Draw back the plunger to fill the syringe with air up to the dose that you need to inject. You need to add an equal amount of air to regulate the pressure. This will make it easier to draw the medication into the syringe (Cafasso 2015).

- You need to push the needle through the rubber stopper at the top of the vial. Inject all the air into the vial (Cafasso 2015).
- Withdraw the medication and remove air bubbles by tapping the syringe to push any bubbles to the top and gently depress the plunger to push the air bubbles out (Cafasso 2015).
- spread the skin at the correct location and insert the needle at a 90-degree angle (except the vastus laterals which requires lifting the muscle) (Craven & Hirnle 2003).
- you need to pull the plunger back slightly. If the blood appears, you need to remove the needle, dispose properly to yellow disposable sharps container and prepare a new injection (Craven & Hirnle 2003).
- You can inject medication slowly if no blood is present while you pull back the plunger slightly (Craven & Hirnle 2003).

If you know the procedure and followed it while practicing, it might give you confidence.

Subcutaneous injection administration

Subcutaneous injection administers under the skin on the fatty tissue or the tissue layer between the skin and muscle (Case-lo 2015). The medication given by this method absorbs more slowly than the medication injected into a vein, sometimes over a period of 24 hours (Case-lo 2015). When other methods of administration are less effective than the subcutaneous method, for example, some medication cannot be given through mouth because enzymes and acid in the stomach would destroy them (Case-lo 2015). Another method such as intravenous injection might be difficult and expensive (Case-lo 2015). For small amounts of delicate drugs administration, the subcutaneous injection can be a useful, safe and convenient method of getting a medication into the human body (Case-lo 2015).

What types of medication can be given subcutaneous?

While administering small volumes, for example, less than 2ml insulin and some hormones are commonly administered as subcutaneous injections (Case-lo 2015).

Some drugs which need to be given very quickly can also be administered via subcutaneous injection (Case-lo 2015). Epinephrine comes in an automated injector or "EpiPen" form that is used to treat severe allergic reactions (Case-lo 2015) quickly. Other pain medications, for example, morphine and hydromorphone can be given subcutaneously as well (Case-lo 2015). Antimatics drugs that prevent nausea and vomiting, for example metoclopramide or dexamethasone, can also be given via subcutaneous injection (Case-lo 2015). Some vaccines and allergy shots are administered as a subcutaneous injection (Case-lo 2015).

The most common injection sites are:

Abdomen: At or under the level of the belly button, approximately two inches away from the navel (Case-lo 2015).

Arm: at the side of the upper arm (Case-lo 2015).

Thigh: front of the thigh (Case-lo 2015).

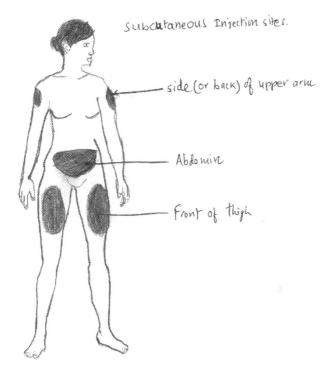

Subcutaneous Injection sites.

— side (or back) of upper arm

— Abdomin

— Front of thigh

(http://www.healthline.com)

Clean and inspect the injection site:

It is always good to inspect the skin to make sure there is no bruising, burns, swelling, hardness or irritation in the area (Case-lo 2015). You need to use alternate injection sites to prevent damage to an area with repeated injections (Case-lo 2015). After that, you should clean the skin with an alcohol swab (Case-lo 2015). Let the area dry before you administer the injection (Case-lo 2015).

How to prepare a syringe?

Remove the cap from the vial: The rubber stopper should be cleaned with an alcohol swab (Case-lo 2015).

Draw air into the Syringe: You need to draw back the plunger to fill the syringe with air up to the dose that you will be injecting into the patient (Case-lo 2015). The reason behind doing this is, the vial is a vacuum, and you need to add an equal amount of air to regulate the pressure (Case-lo 2015). This makes it easier to draw the medication into the syringe (Case-lo 2015). This is one of the easiest ways to draw the medication from a vial (Case-lo 2015).

Insert air into the vial: You need to remove the cap from the needle and push the needle through the rubber stopper at the top of the vial (Case-lo 2015). Now you need to inject all the air into the vial (Case-lo 2015). You need to be very careful to keep the needle aseptic or clean (Case-lo 2015).

Withdraw the medication: You need to turn the vial and syringe upside down so the needle points upward (Case-lo 2015). Then, pull back on the plunger to withdraw the correct amount of medication (Case-lo 2015).

Remove the air bubbles: Tap the syringe to push any bubbles to the top and gently depress the plunger to push the air bubbles out (Case-lo 2015).

Inject the medication

Pinch the skin: You need to pinch the skin between your thumb and index finger and hold it. (Your forefinger and the thumb should be about an inch and a half apart) (Case-lo 2015). This will pull the fatty tissue away from the muscle and makes the injection easier (Case-lo 2015).

Inject the needle: This is important, inject the needle into the pinched skin at a 90-degree angle. You should do this quickly, but without great force (Case-lo 2015). Important, if your patient has very little fat on his body, you may need to inject the needle at a 45-degree angle to the skin (Case-lo 2015).

Insert the medication: slowly push the plunger to inject the medication. You should inject the entire amount of medication (Case-lo 2015).

Withdraw the needle: Let go of the pinched skin and withdraw the needle. Discard the used needle in a puncture- resistant sharp's container (Case-lo 2015).

Apply pressure to the site: Use gauze to apply light pressure to the injection site, if there is any bleeding (Case-lo 2015). You may notice a little bruising later. This is common and nothing to be worried about (Case-lo 2015).

ABCDEFG Assessment
(The systematic Nursing Assessment tool)

The ABCDEFG approach is applicable for all critically ill patients for both children and adults. The ABCDEFG approach should be used whenever critical illness or injury is suspected. It is a valuable tool to identify or rule out critical conditions in daily practice (NSWH 2011).

Before beginning the assessment, first, one's own safety must be ensured. Then the general observation is obtained by simply looking at the patient's skin colour, sweating and surroundings (New South Wales Health (NSWH) 2011).

A – airway: Is the patient's airway patent?

You need to observe the chest wall movement of the patient. Listen for first airway patency for example, if the patient can speak. In this situation, airway is generally okay (NSWH 2011). Signs of a partially obstructed airway may include changed voice, noisy breathing for example strider, gurgling and wheezing may indicate compromised airway (NSWH 2011). A reduced level of consciousness is a common symptom of airway obstruction (NSWH 2011). Untreated airway obstruction can lead to cardiac arrest (NSWH 2011). Head tilt and chin – lift to open the airway. If possible, foreign bodies causing airway obstruction should be removed (NSWH 2011). If the victim becomes unconscious, call for help and start cardiopulmonary resuscitation according to guidelines (NSWH 2011). Importantly, high- flow oxygen should be provided to all critically ill person as soon as possible (New South Wales Health (NSWH) 2011).

B – Breathing:

Count the respiratory rate for 30- 60'

Inspect movements of the thoracic wall for symmetry and use of auxiliary respiratory muscle and percuss the chest for unilateral dullness or resonance. If a stethoscope is available, lung auscultation should be performed and if possible pulse oximeter should be applied (NSWH 2011).

Appearance: diaphoretic, cyanotic, restless/ anxious (NSWH 2011).

Listen: can the patient talk in full sentences, short sentence or words only? (NSWH 2011).

Feel: any tracheal shift, surgical emphysema and swelling (NSWH 2011).

If breathing is insufficient, assisted ventilation must be performed by giving rescue breaths with or without a barrier device. Trained personnel should use a bag mask if available (NSWH 2011).

C – Circulation: Is the patient has circulation sufficient?

Peripheral perfusion: check colour, temperature, capillary refill < 2 secs

- Check if there is any blood loss
- Check the blood pressure
- Feel the pulse (regular/irregular, weak/ strong)
- Does the patient have warm hands and feet? (NSWH 2011).

Hypotension is an important adverse clinical sign. The effects of hypovolemia can be alleviated by placing the patient in the supine position and elevating the patient's legs (NSWH 2011). If this the case, an intravenous access should be obtained as soon as possible and saline should be infused (NSWH 2011).

D – Disability:

Consciousness level of the patient can be assessed using the AVPU method. Where the patient is graded alert (A), voice responsive (V), pain responsive (P) and unresponsive (U) (NSWH 2011). The most important assessment is Glasgow Coma Score (GCS) which can be used (NSWH 2011). Limb movements should be inspected to evaluate the potential of lateralization (NSWH 2011). The best approach to treating the patient with a primary cerebral condition is stabilization of the airway, breathing and circulation (NSWH 2011). When the patient is only pain responsive or unresponsive, airway patency should be ensured by placing the patient in the recovery position. A decreased level of conscious due to low blood glucose can be corrected quickly with oral or infused glucose (NSWH 2011).

E – Exposure

- Check the body temperature
- Skin integrity
- Wounds and drains
- Pain (NSWH 2011).

F – Fluids /food

- Check IV access
- Fluid status – input /output
- Bowels (NSWH 2011).
- Review all charts and documentation
- Nutritional status (NBM, ng tube/feeds? Assistance with meals (NSWH 2011).

G – Glucose

- Blood glucose level monitoring (NSWH 2011).

The ABCDEFG is a strong clinical tool for the initial assessment of patients with acute medical and surgical emergencies, including both pre-hospital first-aid and in- hospital treatment (NSWH 2011).

The use of clinical reasoning cycle, application of critical thinking and coordination of care

While handling a deteriorating patient in a real life situation, it's always going to be challenged at first as a student nurse. When you know how to use critical thinking, and the clinical reasoning cycle correctly and coordination of care, you can handle the challenging situation without a problem and hesitation to achieve the best health outcome. I will give three examples to understand the application of the clinical reasoning cycle, critical thinking and coordination of care in the real clinical setting. These are the examples approved by the hospital's preceptor and clinical facilitator. As a third-year student nurse, you are aiming to utilize the clinical reasoning cycle, critical thinking, and coordination of care while handling a deteriorating patient.

1) Situation, Action, Outcome (SAO)

Situation

One morning, I had a really challenging experience on the busy GIT ward. I was looking after Ms Karma (pseudonym) on a morning shift. She was post-op day 1 and the operation procedure was cholecystectomy. After the medications round, I observed that she was looking pale, looking unwell and was saying that she was feeling weak. I was really worried about her presenting situations. I checked her wound site there was no any ooze or any abnormality. I noticed that something might have gone wrong with her.

Action

Firstly, I did a set of observations on her then checked her previous vital signs record. Her previous blood pressure (BP) was also in lower normal range. I reported it to my preceptor about the situation and informed the vital signs reading. Her blood pressure was 82/59 mmHg, RR 16, HR 95 bpm, SAO2 97 %. And the temperature was 36.4 degree Celsius. My preceptor confirmed my reading by taking manual blood pressure. After that, he contacted the medical team for review. The doctor came within 20 minutes and reviewed her condition and charted 1000mls fluid bolus

IV infusion. Low blood pressures occur because the heart does not have enough blood to pump. Blood loss in the surgery can cause low blood pressure, pulse rate high and urinary output may decrease. To increase the fluid volume in the body, the doctor charted IV fluid bolus. That can help to increase fluid volume in the body and help her to maintain her BP within normal range. If the patient has not got immediate treatment, that could cause hypovolemic shock.

Outcome

After administering the fluid, I went to check her vital signs and her BP was improved 100/80 mmHg. Now, she was feeling better and her medical situations improved through the immediate action taken. IV fluid bolus helped her to maintain fluid in her body and heart to pump the blood normally. The given fluid bolus increased output, organ blood flow restored and arterial blood pressure improved. From this experience, I learnt to respond as quickly as possible to find out what's wrong with the patient and take action for better health outcome.

2) Situation, Action, Outcome (SAO)

Situation

One day, I was looking after Mr. Clark (pseudonym) on a PM shift in the Oncology ward. Mr. Clarke was admitted to the ward on L2 decompression. After the handover when I entered the room I saw him sitting on a chair. I observed that he was trying to lift the bottom part up and trying to lean back and forth. I could clearly observe on his face that he was feeling uncomfortable with pain. I checked his vital signs. They were within normal range. I asked him verbal questions, for example, are you feeling pain? He answered yes, and I asked him about the location of the pain.

He mentioned that he was feeling pain in his back. I was worried about his pain and discomfort.

Action

I conducted a pain assessment. I reported to my preceptor regarding his pain. When I assessed his pain level 0-10 (pain score), 0 is the absence of pain, 1-3 mild pain, 4-6 is moderate pain and 7-10 is the worst possible pain. He mentioned that he was feeling pain on the level of 7 which was the worst possible pain. I looked at his medication chart and found that the doctor had charted PRN Endone. I reported to my preceptor regarding his pain, and she gave him 10 mg Endone via PO. After he had Endone, he settled and I helped him to lie on the bed for rest.

Outcome

After half an hour, I asked him how his pain was. I asked him to rate his pain 0-10. 0 is the absence of pain, 1-3 is mild pain, 4-6 is moderate pain and 7-10 is the worst possible pain. He mentioned that his pain level was about 2. He was settled, and I reassured him that if he felt any pain just let me know. His mobility was unsteady. I also reassured him that if he needed assistance going to the toilet, please press the buzzer and you would be assisted by the nurse. During the shift, the patient compliant. He was assisted in toileting a few times during our shifts and his pain was managed with analgesia with good effect.

3) Situation, Action, Outcome (SAO)

Situation

One day, I was looking after Mr. Jonson (pseudonym) on an AM shift in the Oncology ward. Mr. Jonson was admitted to the ward febrile and tachycardia. His medical history was metastatic prostate cancer. After the handover when I entered the room I saw him sleeping on the bed. I observed that he was looking different than before. He was inactive and looking pale. I checked his vital signs before administering the medication, and the readings were BP 94/61, SPO2 96%, HR 118, RR 16 and temperature 36.1. I noticed that he was hypotensive and tachycardia. I checked his medication chart, and he was in chemotherapy. He was in Abiraterone 1 g daily (hormonal antineoplastic agents).

Action

I reported the vital signs reading to my preceptor, and my preceptor informed the doctor about the patient's current situation regarding hypotension and tachycardia. The doctor charted Hartman 2/24 IV and it was given to the patient immediately. The doctor also charted Hartman 4/24 IV and it was given to the patient after finishing the first IV fluid infusion. I tried to reassure him to eat and drink, but he said to me that he did not feel like eating. The patient might have been hypotensive because of not eating and drinking adequately. If fluid volume decreases in the body, the heart does not have enough blood to pump. Dehydration can cause the patient to be hypotensive, and have tachycardia, and the urine output also may decrease. To increase the fluid volume in the patient's body, the doctor charted IV 2/24 and 4/ 24. That IV fluid infusion helped to increase fluid volume in the body and helped him to maintain his blood pressure within normal range. If the patient did not receive immediate treatment, that might have caused hypovolemic shock.

Outcome

After administering the IV fluid, I went to check his vital signs and his blood pressure was 108/72 mmHg and the heart rate was 98 bpm. Now he was feeling better and his medical situation improved through the action taken. Iv fluid helped him to maintain fluid in his body, and that helped the heart rate to pump blood normally. The given fluid increased output, organ blood flow restored and arterial blood pressure improved. From this experience, I learnt to respond as quickly as possible and identify what's wrong with the patient and take immediate action to achieve the best health outcome.

Respiratory rate

The normal respiratory rate is 10 -20 breaths/minute. The recent evidence suggests that an adult with a respiratory rate of over 20 breaths /minute is probably unwell and an adult with a respiratory rate over 24 breaths/ minute is likely to be critically ill (Cretikos et al. 2008). A raised respiratory rate is a strong and specific predictor of serious adverse events, for example cardiac arrest and unplanned intensive care unit admission (Cretikos et al. 2008). Thus, an adult with a respiratory rate greater than 24 breaths/ minute should be monitored closely and regularly reviewed, even if other vital signs are in within normal range (Cretikos et al. 2008). A patient with a respiratory rate greater than 27 breaths/ minute should receive an immediate medical review (Cretikos et al. 2008).

A patient with a respiratory rate greater than 24 breaths/minute in combination with other evidence of physiological instability, for example, hypotension or a reduced level of consciousness should also receive an immediate medical review (Cretikos et al. 2008).

Some common diseases

Gastrostomy- Abdominal tube going into the stomach. Can be used for feeding or drainage.

Subtotal gastrectomy- Portion of stomach removed.

Total gastrectomy- Complete removal of stomach.

Cholecystectomy- Removal of the gallbladder. Usually done laparoscopically and is mainly due to gallstone.

Hernia- The most common place for a hernia is in the abdomen. Hernias occur when there are weak points in the abdominal wall, and the internal organs start to push out through that point. Common areas to occur are umbilical, inguinal (groin), femoral (just below inguinal) or incisional (occurs at a point of previous surgery) (Farewell & Dempsey 2011).

Whipple's procedure- Surgical procedure to treat ampullary tumours and tumours in the distal common bile duct.

Pancreatitis- Pancreatitis is inflammation of the pancreas. The pancreas is a gland located behind the stomach. It releases the hormones insulin and glucagon as well as digestive enzymes that help you digest and absorb food (Farewell & Dempsey 2011).

Severe acute pancreatitis – may cause dehydration and low blood pressure. The heart, lungs, or kidney can fail. If bleeding occurs in the pancreas, shock, and even death may follow (Farewell & Dempsey 2011). The patient is usually kept NBM to rest the pancreas and given IV fluids; a strict fluid balance chart needs to be managed. Adequate analgesia is essential for abdominal pain and patients are sometimes put on a PCA. IV AB's are administered to treat inflammation (Farewell & Dempsey 2011).

Pseudocytes- It is an accumulation of fluid and tissue debris which may develop in the pancreas and can be drain by using ERCP or EUS. If pseudocysts are left untreated, enzymes and toxins can enter the bloodstream and affect the heart, lungs, kidneys and other organs (Farewell & Dempsey 2011).

Chronic pancreatitis- is the inflammation of the pancreas that does not heal or improve. It gets worse over time and ultimately leads to permanent damage. The most common cause of chronic pancreatitis is many years of heavy alcohol use (Farewell & Dempsey 2011).

Barrett's oesophagus- a condition in which the oesophagus changes. It is closely associated with gastro -oesophageal reflux disease (GORD). Although rare, this can be a precursor to oesophageal cancer.

Mallory – Weiss tear- A tear in the mucous membrane in the lower oesophagus or upper part of the stomach. It is usually caused by long-term vomiting or coughing. The tear can lead to bleeding; however, surgery is rarely required, and the tear will heal in a few days (Farewell & Dempsey 2011).

Oesophageal varices- Varices are distended veins in the oesophagus. Oesophageal varices develop when normal blood flow to your liver is slowed. Varices commonly occur in people with alcoholic liver disease (Farewell & Dempsey 2011).

Oesophagitis- inflammation of the oesophagus.

Oesophagogastrectomy- Performed for cancers in the lower third of the oesophagus. The procedure involves excision of the lower third of oesophagus and the stomach.

Gastritis- Inflammation of gastric mucosa.

Gastric ulcer- erosion in the lining of the duodenum that leads to inflammation and ulceration. 95% of duodenal ulcers are caused by the bacteria Helicobacter Pylori (Farewell & Dempsey 2011).

Peptic Ulcer- erosion in the lining of the stomach or duodenum. Peptic refers to pepsin (stomach enzymes that break down proteins).

Appendicitis- inflammation of the vermiform appendix.

Diverticulitis- Inflammation /infection of the diverticula. Diverticula are small, bulging sacs or pouches of the inner lining of the intestine. Diverticula commonly occur in people who have a low fibre diet (Farewell & Dempsey 2011).

Bowel obstruction- caused by any condition that prevents the normal flow of digestive secretions/ digested food through the intestine. Obstruction can occur due to the following reasons, for example, adhesions, foreign bodies, hernias, volvulus or tumours (Farewell & Dempsey 2011).

Crohn's disease- Crohn's disease causes inflammatory of the full thickness of the bowel wall.

Ulcerative Colitis- Causes inflammation of the inner lining of the large bowel.

Irritable bowel syndrome- IBS affects the nerves and muscles of the bowel.

Colon Polyps- outgrows of the tissue from the wall of the large bowel or colon that vary in size and shape.

Transverse Colectomy- middle of the colon (transverse colon) is removed.

Left hemicolectomy- left side of the colon is removed at the side of the distal transverse.

Sigmoid colectomy (also known as high anterior resection)- removes tumours of the sigmoid colon. The upper rectum and descending colon are anastomosed.

Anterior resection- the sigmoid colon and upper rectum are removed.

Low anterior resection- the mid and low portion of the rectum and above is removed.

Oesophagolaryngectomy- removal of the upper cervical oesophagus and the Larynx.

Maxillectomy- removal of the maxilla and sometimes surrounding bone.

Superficial parotidectomy- removal of the parotid gland with preservation of the facial nerve.

Total Parotidectomy- removal of the parotid gland with the sacrifice of the facial nerve.

Glossectomy- removal of the tongue (can be total/partial /hemi).

Total laryngectomy- Removal of the larynx (voice box), including hyoid bone, cricoid cartilage and 2/3 of the trachea. A permanent tracheal stoma remains for the airway.

Partial laryngectomy- only a portion of the larynx is removed.

Laryngopharyngectomy- removal of the larynx and pharynx.

Total thyroidectomy- removal of the entire thyroid gland.

Partial thyroidectomy- removal of part of the thyroid gland.

Parathyroidectomy- Removal of part or all the parathyroid glands.

Lumpectomy- The tumour is removed, and the major of the breast is left.

Total mastectomy- all breast tissue, including the nipple-areolar complex and the lining over the pectoralis major muscle is removed (Farewell & Dempsey 2011).

These are just examples of the some of the diseases you may encounter in the clinical placement. You also can research about the diseases you encounter in your respective ward and make a list. So, that you can remember, you may also share with your friends. This might be helpful to understand diseases and patients' situations. This will bring confidence to understand the patient's situation.

To master the clinical skill in the clinical placement you need to fully focus on your assigned patient. For example, if you are doing third-year placement, you are assigned four patients. So, focus on the four patients and gather as much information as you can about them from the care plan, doctor's note, operation note, admission note, progress notes. Ask the preceptor if you do not understand anything about your patient. If your patients are cognitively well and communicate well, they will tell you what actually happened to them and how they are managing their disease at the moment and what the doctor is discussing with them, the next treatment plan and procedure. If you ask them, they might actually tell you what's wrong with them and past medical history. I found this method very helpful to understand the patient situation and to promote their health and wellbeing further. That also helps to build trust with the patient between RN. Before going to the PEP, please revise human anatomy and physiology and some terminology. You can also review the abovementioned pharmacology, and you can research the important pharmacology per your placement area for example oncology, GIT, orthopaedic, urology. Use a hand diary to note the disease you encounter and pharmacology. Write them and research about it and try to memorise and understand so that it helps you to administer medication with confidence and safely.

In patient's handover sheet, you may find the following type of examples

BED, MRN, NAME, Sex, AGE, Admin time, Doctor, unit, Alerts,

comments

Nursing: PP: SBO, lethargy

Nursing: 4. Cares: NBM, IVT/PCA (M), NGT-FD & 4/24 ASP, Anti-emetics-palliative

Nursing: 2. PHx: stage 4 Rectal CA (colostomy), Peritoneal and liver metastasis, Prev paracentesis OCT 14, Prev SBO OCT'14

The above handover sheet mentioned in short form of the medical terms. It needs to be understood correctly. Below is the example of what was mentioned above.

Presenting problem: small bowel obstruction and lethargy

There are 4 nursing cares involved as per the handover sheet, these are to summarize patient is nil by mouth, has IV transfusion, patient control analgesia, morphine continue, the patient has nose gastric tube -feed and 4ᵗʰ hourly aspiration required and the patient has anti-emetics medication, and he is in palliative.

Past medical history: stage 4 rectal cancers and using colostomy, he had peritoneal and liver metastasis, previous paracentesis in October 2014, previous small bowel obstruction in October 2014. For example, I did not know the meaning of paracenthasis, so I researched and found out that it means a procedure during which fluid from the abdomen is removed through a needle. Now I completely understand what's wrong with the patient, his medical history, and his care needs clearly.

This is one of the examples of a handover sheet of one patient. There are a lot of short forms and terminology may be used. You need to understand them for your assigned patient. If you do not understand, you may ask the preceptor and facilitator, and you may research them to understand. This brings you confidence about what needs to be done for the patient. Anything you did not understand underline it and find the information as soon as possible for your assigned patient. So, now you are a proactive student nurse and always use a shift planner for time management and prioritise the care of your patients. This shows that you are a serious student seeking the learning opportunities that may impress the preceptor and the facilitator by your attitude. If you are not sure, never guess the answer. Always tell them I will research about it and tell them after. Always respect and act ethically with the preceptor and facilitator and to other health care teams. **I wish you good luck to your PEP.**

New graduate nursing interview preparation

Karma Yoga

I like to experiment with the knowledge and wisdom I hear and read. In my new graduate nursing interview, I experimented about Karma yoga which I studied to lift myself up and back again to my studies. In the book, Gita, Lord Krishna told Arjun to do the action which is required but don't expect the outcome. You only need to concentrate on what you can do, and you should not think and worry about the outcome. Because there is no control of the outcome in your hands. By exactly following Lord Krishna's advice, Arjun fought in the war and won one of the great wars in the history called Mahabharat almost 5000 years ago. His opposition was also a great warrior and powerful; even his guru, Dronacharya, fought against him. In the war, before fighting with all the great warriors and his loved ones, for example Vishma pitamaha (grandfather) and Guru, Arjun was shaking and scared about the outcome, but the Lord Krishana motivated Arjun to fight in the great war to establish dharma and justice for the people. Lord Krishana told Arjun to perform the right action without worrying about any outcome. Krishan said leave it to me whatever happens. Don't worry about the outcome. He believed Krishna's advice and only concentrated on what he could do; this meant focusing on fighting with his arrows. The concept of karma yoga is described as a way of acting, thinking and willing by which one orients oneself towards realization by acting in accordance with one's duty (dharma) without consideration of personal self -centered desires, likes or dislikes. One acts without being attached to the results of one's deeds. It simply means one does not get emotionally involved in the action being performed, becoming overly excited, upset or angry when the result of a deed is not as expected. The result may be negative or positive. Krishna explains to Arjun in the book, Gita, that work done without selfish expectations purifies one's mind and gradually makes an individual fit to see the value of reason. Therefore, without being attached to the results of activities, one should act as a matter of duty, for by working without attachment one attains the supreme.

In the case of the new graduate nursing interview, I utilized the wisdom of karma yoga according to the book, Gita, and concluded that there were two parts which I could put my whole effort of action. It is all in the mind when we start to think our karma starts. So, we have two choices to start karma; either we start to think what action we can carry out and the second we can think about the outcome (results). According to Lord Krishna, outcome is not in your control and it is not even necessary that the outcome should be in your favour. So, I have no right to control the outcome. For me, it was as soon as possible and necessary to understand that I have no control over whatever outcome comes. So, the only option for me is to act on my own action which is 100% in my control. So, I thought deeply about what action I could carry out; I figured out that to enhance my interview I needed to find out what types of question they asked in the interview and thoroughly prepare those questions. Now, my total concentration went to finding out the questions and preparation on them instead of thinking about the outcome. At that point, I completely detached from the outcome which was not in my control. When I did that, I became fearless and freed from the attachment to the outcome. My whole focus went on their questions and how I was going to answer them. My brain was freed from thinking regarding outcome pass or fail and success or being unsuccessful. I was focused to hit the exact target of their questions through my answers. My brain already expected their questions and as ready to response with the exact answer they expected from me. The only thing that matters is their question and my answer and nothing else. If their questions and my answers matched and meet their expectation, this would increase my possibility of getting the job. If their questions and my answers did not match and did not meet their expectations, I would have less possibility to have a positive outcome. So my focus should be to respond to their questions as they expected to be right. The answers I needed to tell them should be right and meet their expectations. There would be three interviewers, and they would write notes and mark my answer. So, I needed to give my answers to them at a normal pace (speed) so they could write my answers and I needed to speak with clear pronunciation so that they could understand what I told them. I thought and acted the way I described before, and I believe this strategy of karma yoga helped me to secure a new graduate nursing position.

The Interview Process

Interview preparation is vital, and you need to check the interview process and questions criteria with the advertiser. It may change so, please check them. You must read the position description and be aware of what the role entails. All questions in the interview relate to the criteria of the position. Here is some information about the interview process.

There are 6 questions asked in the interview. They all relate to the essential criteria of the position.

The panel will consist of 3 members who will ask 2 questions each; each panel member's score is then added together to give your final total score.

The following themes are commonly referred to at the transition to professional practice interviews:

- Personal and professional skills and attributes -what you can personally and professionally contribute to the ward and organization.

- conflict resolution scenario- what would you do in the situation? How would you handle it?
- communication and teamwork- What makes it work? The ability to work in interdisciplinary team
- scope of practice and legislation, e.g., work health and safety, competency standard of the RN, infection control
- Scenario-based question where you need to prioritise care using a structured assessment process, e.g. DETECT, A-G assessment.
- CORE values of NSW Health and how you apply them to practice with example demonstration.

You need to answer the questions giving examples where possible to demonstrate your experience. Be clear and concise in your answers.

Try to answer the questions as if you are the RN in the situation, not as a student.

Preparation for interview

- Remember you never get a second chance to make a good first impression.
- Remember practice makes man perfect, so practice well so that you are ready for the answers.
- Excellent communication skill and speaking with the examples would show your understanding around the questions asked in the interview that may differentiate you from another candidate.
- Bring all the information required, for example, documents for 100-point ID check and other required documentation and health card.
- Arrive early for the interview because you may need to park your car and you may need to show all the required

documents to the counter before the interview. I prefer that you come earlier so you do not have any rush.

- Dress professionally. Choose the dress which can show your personality.
- Wear your hair up as if you are doing a shift.
- Give eye contact; look at the person asking the question.
- Be confident.
- Smile.
- Please answer truthfully.
- Ask for question to be repeated if you do not understand.
- If you are asked something in the interview after the question, they already asked this can be a sign you may have gone off track, or they may prompt you for more information.
- You can always ask to go back to a question if you think of something else.
- At the end of the interview, they may give you a chance to ask questions of them and the information you may want to know from them. If you have the question you may ask them.

During my new graduate nursing interview, I prepared some of the questions which helped me to enhance my interview preparation that also helped me to secure the new graduate nursing position. I gathered some questions from friends and researched myself. Here are some of the questions you can also practice to enhance your interview process. Always be open-minded and ask another friend as well how they are preparing and share your ideas as well.

The new graduate nursing job interview questions types with answers

1) What are the roles and responsibilities of a registered nurse? Can you please explain?

According to the ANMC competency standard, registered nurse role and responsibilities are as follows:

- The registered nurse demonstrates competence in the provision of nursing care as specified by the registering authority's licence to practice, educational preparation, relevant legislation, standards of codes and context of care (Nursing and Midwifery Board of Australia (NMBA) 2006)
- The registered nurse practices independently and interdependently assuming accountability and responsibility to their own actions and delegation of care to enrolled nurses and health care workers (NMBA 2006). Delegation takes into consideration the education and training of enrolled nurses and health care workers and the context of care (NMBA 2006).
- The registered nurse provides evidence-based nursing care to people of all ages and cultural groups, including individuals, families, and communities (NMBA 2006).
- The role of the registered nurse includes promotion and maintenance of health and prevention of illness for individuals with physical and mental illness, disabilities and or rehabilitation needs, as well as alleviation of pain and suffering at the end stage of life (NMBA 2006).
- The registered nurse assesses, plans, implements and evaluates nursing care in collaboration with individuals and the multidisciplinary health care team to achieve goals and health outcomes (NMBA 2006).
- The registered nurse recognizes that ethnicity, culture, gender, spiritual values, sexuality, age, disability and economic and social factors have an effect on an individual response to, and beliefs about, health and illness and plans and modifies nursing care appropriately (NMBA 2006).

- The registered nurse provides care in a range of setting, for example, acute, community, residential, and extended care settings, homes, educational institutions and other work settings and modifies practice according to the models of care delivery (NMBA 2006).

- The registered nurse takes a leadership role in the coordination of nursing and health care within and across different care contexts to facilitate optimal health outcome (NMBA 2006). This may include appropriate referral to, and consultations with, other relevant health professionals, service providers and community and support services (NMBA 2006).

- The registered nurse contributes to quality health care through professional development and lifelong learning himself/herself and others, research data generation, clinical practice guidelines and clinical supervision and development of policy (NMBA 2006).

- The registered nurse develops their professional practice in accordance with health needs of the population/ society and changing patterns of disease and illness (NMBA 2006).

2) What are your professional and personal qualities that will contribute to the hospital? Or what skills can you bring to our organization?

Or

You are a new member of the nursing profession what personal and professional qualities do you bring to the nursing team?

Some of the professional and personal qualities that will contribute to the hospital are as follows. You can add more if you have any additional qualities.

Communication

- Clear concise written and verbal communication within the multidisciplinary team
- Utilize active listening skills to hear the concerns of the patient
- Keep the patient and significant others informed of health care and plan of care and maintain communication with multidisciplinary team
- Introduce self at the beginning of the shift to build rapport and trust with the patient
- Introduce self and procedures to patients and significant others

Ensure safe practice and priority of patient safety first

- The primary role of the Australian health practitioner's regulation agency (AHPRA) is to protect the public.
- As a registered nurse, I will practice safely within the healthcare environment and will maintain patient safety. To ensure safe practice and patient safety before administering the medication I will conduct the five rights and checks, for example, the right patient, the right drug, the right dose, the right route, and the right time. I also will check whether the patient has any known allergy history and the expiry of the medication to be used. I will sign and document.
- utilization of critical thinking and analysis to achieve the best health outcome
- I will use the clinical reasoning cycle to conduct the comprehensive nursing assessment
- I will use the ISBAR (introduction, situation, background, assessment and recommendation) communication tool to

communicate with the doctors effectively for the safety of the patient and to achieve the best health outcome.

- For the safety of the patient, I will follow clinical guidelines, hospital policy and protocols and drug reference guidebook, for example MIMS and Australian injectable drugs handbook.

Respect patient's privacy, dignity, confidentiality and cultural preferences

- Respect the autonomy of patients in active participation in health care
- Respect their cultural differences and choices
- Drawing curtains for privacy and use of dignity gown to maintain their dignity

Punctuality

- Always on time if not early to ensure handover can take place and previous shift may leave on time. Maintains morale and collegiality

Presentation skills

- Can use presentation skill to educate patients, colleagues and significant others

Organization skills

- Can organize the task, time management, delivery the task timely manner and documentation

Research skills

- Conduct evidence-based research to treat the patient and formulate research-based practices
- Help inform and develop the policy

Collegiality

- Teamwork and team cohesion are significant in providing optimal holistic care
- Help to improve morale, rapport and team cohesion maintaining productivity and efficacy

Sense of Humour

- Handle the job pressure calmly
- Handle conflict management and resolve the problem by addressing appropriately
- Utilization of self-reflection to improve self
- Help other colleagues while required any assistance

3) What skill do you have which is suited to the registered nurse?

You can talk about your graduate attributes (personal and professional)

- Delivered patient centred care in a professional, competent manner
- Utilize communication and collaboration skill
- Prioritize care
- Time management
- Work-life balance

- Caring for the patient, promote holistic care, health and well-being

4) What is mean by an interdisciplinary team? How do you work in an interdisciplinary team? Explain with examples.

The interdisciplinary team involves a group of health care professionals for diverse fields who work in a coordinated fashion toward a common goal for the patient. For example, for patients, it improves care by increasing coordination of services, especially for complex problems. A patient can get a variety of services and treatment in one place for instance physiotherapy, dietician, social worker, physician, and specialist doctor. It also empowers patients as an active partner in care and uses time more efficiently.

- For registered nurses and other health care professionals, it helps to increase professional satisfaction. It also enables them to learn new skills, approaches, innovation and focuses on a particular expertise area. In an interdisciplinary team, individual goals are set, and each discipline works to achieve the goal within the scope of practice, for example, doctors, registered nurses, physio and social workers all work to achieve health goal and wellbeing of the patient. In the interdisciplinary team, all the individuals have their individual goals and to achieve that goal they need to work together as a team.

5) Discovery that an anti-hypertensive had not been given for three days

- Initial reaction: Surprise (used humour and true portrayal of self which convenor's appreciated)

115

- Ask patient whether he had medication or not, check medication chart, and check documentation for example progress notes
- Take full set of obs (if out of flags may be R/V or MET/PACE call)
- If out of flags, doctor may prescribe antihypertensive transdermal patch, therefore monitor BP and risk of orthostatic hypotension.
- After R/V follow doctor's order and re-administer when indicated.
- **Document:** especially name, dose, and route and location of the patch.

6) Explain what to do if asked to leave a prepared injection oral medication unsupervised.

- Refuse (The reason behind this practice is open to the risk of the following)
- Contamination
- Potential instability
- Potential mix up
- Threatens the security of the medication

7) What is the correct course of action if the drug administration error occurs?

- Take observation of patient vital signs
- Inform NIC, NUM, MO, patient and their person for notification
- Document in the patient's notes
- Complete IIMS

8) What do you do if the prescriber assured you that an unusually high medication was okay to administer?

- Inform NIC
- Consult with colleagues
- Consult with MO
- Consult with Pharmacist
- Look in the MIMS for correct doses

9) Who can carry S4 and S8 drug Keys?

- RNs only carry S8 and S4 drug keys but not together
- NIC or delegated RN carries S8 drug keys
- EENs can carry S4 drug keys only

There is always a scenario question. This type of question is all about knowing your limitations, prioritizing, delegation and getting your team involved. In prioritizing care, think about your colleagues and how your team can help. When answering questions, tell the panel why you would prioritize that way.

For example, you may start your talk; this patient gets my attention first because…"

This patient can wait because…"

This shows critical thinking and clinical skills

10) The scenario given as an example was: There are three patients, diabetic hypo, aggressive patient and chest pain. How would you prioritize the care of three patients?

You need to acknowledge at first that you are unable to deal with all three and **call for help from your team.**

Prioritize—acknowledge that you may need **further information.** For example, what is the **BSL** of the patient?

Potentially, **the chest pain** can be life-threatening, and you need to delegate the other patients to the rest of the team.

You need to assess the urgency of the chest pain and the urgency of the hypo whether **the patient is conscious or not.** Remember, it is a cardiac unit ruled out. Therefore, **assessments are a priority here.** The **BSL and LOC of the hypo patient may mean that they are the priority.**

The **aggressive patient may be settled** with reassurance, and another member of the team may assist him to calm down. First, need to find out his concerns. For example, has he got dementia? Is there any mental health issue? Does he want to go toilet? Is he in pain? if unable to settle can doctor help? If totally violent in this situation may need security.

Show them how you are critically thinking and why you are thinking that way. You may mention the vital signs of the patient and acknowledge the between the flags as well.

11) One patient BSL 2.8, fluids require to change the second patient, the third patient complaining chest pain, how would you prioritize the care of three patients?

Example demonstration

I will attend the chest pain because chest pain can be life-threatening to the patient. That is why he/she needs immediate treatment. I will ask for help from another team member to attain and monitor the level of consciousness of the hypoglycaemic patient. Let the IV pump 'beep', as it will alert another team member to attend to it while we are prioritising care.

Chest pain

- Alcohol based hand rub or hand hygiene
- Draw the curtains for privacy
- ABCD (explain each, for instance, airway, breathing, circulation and disability)
- Describe pain, for instance, location, scale 1-10, ask if had this kind of pain before
- Full obs (may be a MET if far out of limits)
- ECG (assessing PQRST)
- Inform doctor / in-charge

Proceed with treatment with doctor (some hospital policy is to give ½ an anginine tablet sublingual and then the other half 2-5 minutes if pain persists) or per clinical guidelines of chest pain provided by the hospital policy.

- **Document**

BSL- Hypoglycaemic

- Alcohol based hand rub/ hand hygiene
- Draw the curtains for privacy
- ABCD (explain each, for instance, airway, breathing, circulation and disability)
- Recheck BSL; ask if diabetic/ last eaten
- Food/lollies/ hypo-kit
- Full obs
- Notify doctor / in-charge
- Postprandial BSL @ 15, 30, 45 and 60 mins to monitor
- Document

IV Fluids

- Alcohol based hand rub or hand hygiene
- Draw the curtains
- Stop machine
- Check IV site (phlebitis, infection, patency)
- Check order
- Get stock
- Verify order with another registered nurse
- Prepare/ disconnect the previous one
- Clean the cannula
- Connect
- Check
- Run
- **Document**

12) Discovery of patient on shower floor with haemorrhaging head trauma

DRSABCD (check for danger, responsive -ask name and squiz, send for help and call 000, check airway, breathing (look, listen and feel), start CPR and apply a defibrillator.

If no pulse, call a MET and start CPR

Once the team arrives, remove from the shower, and place the patient on dry linen/ towels/ sheets and then proceed to attach defibrillator.

Document

Think of placing a patient with closely monitoring and put patient afterwards with hourly obs.

Possible infection control questions

13) A patient is sent from ED for admissions with gastro and vomiting. How do you manage this patient?

Example answer: I will isolate the patient and will use appropriate PPE and door signage. Personal protective equipment (PPE) is anything used to worn by a person to minimise a risk to their health or safety. I would want him to have his own toilet for infection control reason and for the safety of the other patients. I would check to see if a sample has been sent or needs to be collected. I will check whether the patient has fluid orders and medication such as antiemetic. If the patient does not have any order, I will contact the doctor. I will also inform the infection control staff.

Ethical, procedural question

14) You are checking an S8 with another RN, and she is called away. She asks you to give it, and she will sign later.

Example answer: Ask the RN to commit to the task first before leaving. As a registered nurse, I am fully aware that New South Wales poison and therapeutic goods act and poison and therapeutic goods regulation detect that New South Wales health policies and health directives regarding S8 medication clearly state that two registered nurses who remove the drug from the drug cupboard must then be taking that drug to the patient together and both nurses need to sign the medication chart after administering the prescribed dose and after conducting five rights.

The law states that the same 2 nurse must be involved in the giving of the S8, otherwise it is against law, policy and procedure.

This type of activity may put a patient and staff at risk.

Let the RN know that she needs to come with you. If she refuses and the medication has been dispensed, then you need to talk to the NUM (Nurse Unit Manager) as the medication needs to be destroyed once dispensed.

You need to be able to solve the problem and educate the RN on what is right and appropriate. Use negotiation skills.

NSW health staff members are required to report all identified clinical incidents, near misses and complaints in the state-wide Incident Information Management System (IIMS). It is one of the world's largest clinical incident reporting systems (http://www.cec.health.nsw.gov.au/programs/patient-safety). IIMS may be needed if the RN would not commit the policy and procedure.

Work health and safety related question

15) Your colleague wants to lift a patient without and appropriate lifting device. What would you do?

You need to suggest to the colleague a safer way of lifting the patient. Follow the manual handling policy. You need to check the care plan regarding patient's mobility and transfer. If you check that care plan, you can clearly identify what sorts of device the patient needs to transfer. So please check that first before you start lifting the patient. For example, in the care plan you can find the following:

- **Weight Bearing**: nil, partial, full
- **Mechanical Lifter**: yes, no
- **Mobility**: assist, supervise, independent
- **Mobility aids**: Pelican Belt, etc.

If in the patient's care plan it is stated that a mechanical lifter is required, then you both need to use the mechanical lifter to lift the patient. If your colleague wants to lift a patient without the mechanical lifter in this situation, you should say no. You need to explain and show your colleague the patient's care plan. If he still forces you to lift the patient without a lifting device, you should say no to him and report it to the NUM (Nurse Unit Manager). All staffs are bound to follow the manual handling policy. So, you just need to follow the care plan. What the care plan says and you need to follow your health care's manual handling policy.

16) First time conducting a procedure

- Plan ahead at the beginning of the shift and locate a preceptor/ educator
- Inform the team leader of first time and that you have arranged a preceptor
- Arrange a mutual time for procedure with patient and preceptor
- Check the policy and clinical guidelines
- As nearing time, collect instruments and check preceptor if he or she is ready
- May need to help preceptor with making time (ask if they would like their obs/toileting done on patients to make time for procedure- transactional leadership)
- Make sure to ensure hand hygiene of you and preceptor before the procedure and after.
- **Document**

17) MRSA Patient /Infection control

- Ensure appropriate signs are displayed, and PPE is available
- Wash hands prior (5 moments of hand hygiene)

- PPE as per policy
- Dispose of PPE immediately as leaving the room
- Alcohol based hand rub immediately, then proceed to wash hands
- Ensure PPE is restocked
- **Document**
- Educate patient, significant others, allied health on importance of infection control (importance of 5 moments of hand hygiene)
- Ensure PPE is always restocked PRN
- Use of poster onwards
- Partake in infection control audits
- 5 moments of hand hygiene
- Alcohol based hand rub

18) Discovery of med in patient room

- If there is no nurse in the room, dispose of in sharps (as you do not know what medication is in the cup, putting down the drain may increase the global antibiotic resistance if one of the medicines is an antibiotic).
- Review medication chart, ask patient and check documentation
- Check with assigned RN /EN if available
- Inform team leader and re-administer
- **Document**

19) How do you handle aggressive patient?

- One of the most important steps you can take when confronting an aggressive patient is to remain calm.
- Someone who is acting angry may simply be frightened, defensive or resistant to what is going on around them. It is important for the nurse to take a step back from the

patient who is angry and ask herself what is really going on. The best cause of action is to carefully interview the patient to draw out what they are feeling.

- Use reflective statements, such as, 'I can understand how you feel that way', and try to discuss a possible solution with them.
- Speak softly and refrain from having a judgemental attitude.
- Try to remain neutral, although it may be difficult with an irrational patient.
- Put some distance between yourself and the patient, and do not make intense eye contact. This could set them off.
- You also should try to demonstrate control of the situation without becoming demanding or authoritative.
- See if any of the staff have a rapport with the patient who may be able to calm the situation.
- Ask / determine the reason for being upset and try to resolve the issue from the root rather than pacifying.
- May need to alert security to attend the ward, but remain out of view.
- **Document**

Infection prevention and control

Standard precaution- are meant to reduce the risk of transmission of bloodborne and other pathogens from both recognized and unrecognized sources (WHO 2007). They are a basic level of infection control precautions which are to be used, as a minimum, in the care of all patients (WHO 2007). In addition to hand hygiene, personal protective equipment should be used for standard precaution. Personal protective equipment for example, gloves, aprons, gown, mask, eyewear can be used as a standard precaution in the health care setting (WHO 2007).

20) Can you tell me about transmission -based percussions? How do you look after the patient who has transmitted disease? This question is very important in infection control section.

Transmission-Based Precaution- used in addition to standard precautions when managing patients suspected or known to be being infected with particular agents transmitted by the contact, droplet or airborne routes (DHHS 2014).

There are three types of transmission-based precautions: these are as follows.

Contact Transmission: The diseases spread by direct or indirect contacts are in this category. Patients/ residents which have an infection that can be spread by direct or indirect contact with the person's skin, faeces, mucous membranes, urine, vomit, wound drainage or other body fluids or due to contact with equipment or environmental surfaces that may be contaminated by the patient or resident or due to his/ her secretions and exertions (Department of Health and Human Services (DHHS) 2014)

Contact transmission examples are scabies, salmonella, shigella and pressure ulcers.

Contact precautions:
In addition to standard precaution

- Single-patient room. Ensuite preferred.
- Wear a gown and gloves upon room entry of a patient / resident on contact precaution.
- Remove gown/ apron and gloves and perform hand hygiene after leaving the room (DHHS 2014).
- Use disposable single-use equipment such as blood pressure cuffs and stethoscopes.

- Transmission-based disease, for example clostridium difficile and norovirus special contact precaution are required.

Droplet transmission: Patient/residents that have an infection which can be spread through close respiratory or mucous membrane contact with respiratory secretions (DHHS 2014).

Droplet precaution: In addition to standard precaution

- Single-patient room. Ensuite preferred.
- Conditions that require droplet precaution are influenza, N. meningitides, pertussis (whooping cough), and rhinovirus (known as common cold).
- In addition to standard precaution, wear a surgical mask upon room entry of the patient on droplet precautions and dispose of the mask after leaving the room and perform hand hygiene (DHHS 2014).
- Limit patient movement outside the room to medically-necessary purposes.
- Patient to put on a surgical mask when leaving the room.

Airborne Transmission: fine airborne particles containing infective agents are dispersed over long distances by air and can be inhaled by susceptible persons (DHHS 2014).

Airborne precaution: In addition to standard precaution

- Single negatively pressured room with ensuite.
- Door to remain closed.
- Conditions that require airborne precautions are chicken pox, measles, and tuberculosis.
- To the standard precautions, wear a N95/P2 mask prior to room entry, depending on the disease-specific recommendation. Remove and dispose of the mask and

perform hand hygiene after leaving the room (DHHS 2014).

- When possible, non- immune health care worker should not care for patients with vaccine preventable airborne disease (such as measles and chicken pox).
- Instruct patient about respiratory hygiene and cough etiquette.
- Patient to put surgical mask when leaving the room.

21) As a registered nurse you will be working in a team environment typically you may be caring for the following three patients.

One patient has IV antibiotic due at 1400 and it's already 1430 pm. Another patient complaining of feeling very weak and light-headed. The third patient with a history of high blood pressure and he has a nose bleed. Can you tell the panel how you will prioritise care of three patients and why?

As I am working in a team as a registered nurse in a hospital setting in Australia, I would ask for assistance from another nurse from the team to conduct an assessment of the patient with a nose bleed. I will attend the patient complaining of feeling very weak and light-headed. I would prioritise to address this patient first because he may be experiencing presyncope state and early intervention would require to prevent him from fainting. I would reposition the light-headed patient to supine position and obtain a full set of vital signs and conduct A -G assessment.

I would inform the team member available to help the patient with nose bleed has a history of hypertension. He might be having an episode of hypertension so, I would request to team member to obtain a full set of vital signs and complete A-G assessment and note any of the deterioration.

I would ask another team member if she is not handling unstable patient to commence IV antibiotic. As I am aware that antibiotic is already due and the dose and timing are important. I would not move to this patient until my other patient stabilizes.

22) I would like you to give four examples, and you need to prioritise the four patients.

The first patient has a medication due. The second patient has a cannula tissue. The third patient is verbally aggressive, and the fourth patient has oxygen saturation at 88%. Can you please explain to the panel how you prioritise care for these four patients and why?

The patient with oxygen saturation at 88% is the immediate concern. This patient requires immediate oxygen therapy by Hudson mask at 6 lt. This patient is clinically deteriorating, and I would not leave this patient until the management plan is implemented.

I would call for help from another member of the team to assess the verbally aggressive patient. As I am aware that changing mood of the patient can be the sign of decreasing mental state and hypoxia and the deterioration needs to be assessed. This patient should not be left alone until the management plan is implemented.

The patient with a tissued cannula is the risk of further damage unless the IV is ceased immediately and removed. I would ask another member of the team to do that and assess the patient condition and infusion type. The priority of this patient is to get the cannula replaced as soon as possible.

The patient with medication due cannot be forgotten. I would ask another member of the team to distribute the medication while I attend the other patient. If the medication is time critical, for example insulin, I would insist on gaining help from another member of the team to give the insulin on time.

23) An understanding of the professional, ethical and legal requirement of the registered nurse or registered midwife.

Registered nurses must practice within professional, legal and ethical responsibilities. They must demonstrate that they have a satisfactory knowledge, take accountability and must work in accordance with legislation. They must comply with relevant legislation, common law and duty of care. They must follow the code or professional conduct and code of ethics. They must practice in a safe and competent manner. They must respect dignity, culture, ethnicity, values and beliefs of their patients. They must treat all information confidentially and provide honest and accurate information in relation to nursing care. They must provide informed decision making and promote and preserve the trust and privilege within the nurse-patient relationship. They should respect the patient. They must value diversity, informed decision making and develop a culture of safety in nursing and health care. They must value a social, economically sustainable environment promoting health and wellbeing.

24) Can you tell the panel what you understand about equal employment opportunity mean and can you give an example how it will be implemented in the health care setting?

Equal Employment Opportunity (EEO) is making sure that everyone has equal access to available employment by ensuring that workplaces are free from discrimination and harassment and providing programs to assist people to overcome disadvantage.

That includes having workplace rules, policies, practices, and behaviours that are fair and do not disadvantage people.

For example, this means that the best applicant will be selected following an objective and thorough assessment of an applicant's suitability in relation to the selection criteria of registered nurses.

25) What do you understand about occupational health and safety (OHS) in the workplace mean?

Occupational health and safety (OHS) refers to legislation, policics, procedures and activities that aim to protect the health, safety and welfare of all people at the workplace. For example, manual handling policy and procedure in the hospital.

26) NSW health strives to reflect CORE values in the workplace. What is your understanding of what the C represents? Please give an example.

The code of conduct outlines an ethical and professional framework for those who work as part of NSW health are expected to work within the core values. These CORE values are collaboration, openness, respect, and empowerment. These values will facilitate the possible work culture and one of the main reasons I wish to secure employment in such a community where I can contribute and promote health and well-being by implementing NSW CORE values in day to day practice. The workplace culture framework has been designed to embed cultural improvement strategies as part of the core business in every facility (NSWDH 2011).

The workplace culture framework embodies CORE values: collaboration, openness, respect, and empowerment.

Collaboration

Under NSW health we work collaboratively with each other to achieve the best possible outcomes for our patients who are at the centre of everything we do (NSWDH 2011). While working collaboratively, we acknowledge that every member of the team working in the health system plays a valuable role that contributes to achieving the best possible outcome (New South Wales Department of Health (NSWDH) 2011). For example, holistic care is a team effort, and no single profession can achieve holistic care solely. While assessing the patient throughout the care we need to consider the patient's needs; for example, a psychologist may be needed if there are psychological issues to the patient and a dietician may be required if the patient needs a dietary plan to be implemented.

Collaboration and example demonstration

One male patient had joined the diabetes and metabolic rehabilitation centre clinic previously but recently ceased to continue and gained weight after his father passed away. Some of the team were sceptical that the patient would remain engaged in the clinic appointments. It was a collaborative effort (doctor, dietician, psychologist, exercise therapist, endocrinologist) to discuss his eligibility to re-join the clinic of which all aspects of the patient were considered.

Openness and example demonstration

NSW health encourages the community to have confidence in their local health services. Through open communication, it can foster cooperation and confidence between the team members (NSWDH 2011). For example, openness in the workplace can be established through feedback from the patients and employees. It can be obtained through surveys. It takes feedback as a great tool to improve (NSWDH 2011).

For example, we were two registered nurses going to perform a complex wound dressing for a patient. One RN is preparing the dressing equipment and sterile field. She unintentionally contaminated the sterile field and did not notice it. I noticed the sterile field was contaminated due to a mistake which was a threat to patient safety if the sterile field was not maintained 100 percent. So, I told her that she mistakenly contaminated the sterile field. She welcomed my feedback immediately, and I went to collect the new dressing pack. We re- prepared and did the dressing. Through openness in communication, we achieved patient safety and job satisfaction to both of us as well.

Respect and example demonstration

NSW health considers patients' fundamental rights to be treated with dignity, compassion, and respect. For example, it can be implemented by listening to the patient voice and concerns (NSWDH 2011). It respects all the employees and their rights. It welcomes their contributions. It enhances and makes all the employees responsible for workplace culture and performance. It discourages bullying in the workplace (NSWDH 2011).

In the workplace, NSW health respects the patients' choices and preferences. For example, a food delivery person distributed non-vegetarian food to one of my patients. The patient told me that he does not like to eat non- vegetarian food. He told me that he was vegetarian. In that situation, I respected his choices and preferences and provided vegetarian food per his preferences. In that situation, I respected his choices and preferences in an appropriate manner.

Empowerment and example demonstration

NSW health supports local decision making and innovation with accountability. It provides resources to meet patients' and communities' expectation (NSWDH 2011). Under NSW health, all the professionals are empowered to make the difference in the workplace (NSWDH 2011). Patients are also empowered to ask for information and voice their concern. NSW health strives for individual excellence on behalf of patients on the team to deliver the best possible care and services (NSWDH 2011).

Registered nurses are empowered to use critical thinking on their own thought process and can utilize the tools of the clinical reasoning cycle to make the clinical decision to achieve the best health outcome for the patient. For example, the patient is feeling severe pain (8/10). In this situation, a registered nurse can ask the doctor for immediate review to administer analgesia for the patient's pain management.

Patient empowerment means they can ask doctors questions and concerns regarding their treatment process. They can also appoint family or relatives to help sort through all the information. They are empowered to choose the treatment options suitable for each individual. The patient is given the authority to negotiate on nursing care schedule, for example, time for bed making, showering and what activities to take part in. The patient will be informed before a procedure is performed. Patients are encouraged to make decisions on their own care.

At the End

Even if you faced challenges and difficulties, you can get through it. You will achieve your dreams if you pursue them consistently. Human life is unique. If one door is closed, another door would open for you. You just need to be ready for that and accept the reality and then you will find the solution. It is my personal experience that throughout the journey of my life many doors were closed to me. When the doors were closed, I got upset as well because it's human nature. Now, I thank God that some doors were closed and some were delayed; that was good for me. Some doors opened that were better than the closed ones. I also would like to thank God for that as well. I love the Lord Krishna's philosophy that if things happened to me as I wanted it to be is good and if it did not happen to me as I wanted, it is even better for me. In fact, throughout my journey of my life, it was 100% true to me up to now. We as human beings hold the great power which is the power of choice that belongs to us each moment of our life. You can choose what you think and how you feel. You certainly become what you choose to be. The moment you hold the power of choice, I believe you all become what you choose to be. In reality, while perusing your dream, some doors may close, and some will delay opening. Thanks to God, the door closed for you. Learn from the experience and move on to next one. Life is not any destination that you reach and stop forever; rather, it's a journey. What matters in the journey is move on by learning from the experiences. When you learn from your experiences (practical) combined with knowledge (theory and wisdom), you will become an expert. When you become an expert, thousands of doors will open for you, and you can choose the great one. I believe you all are born to win and succeed.

While I was in my last clinical placement, my preceptor was a clinical nurse specialist. I worked with her almost in total one week; she was friendly, and her style of teaching was very effective. She suggested us to keep three things in mind while doing the new graduate nursing program. Always be committed to doing safe practice, prioritization of care and time management. Always ask to other staff members if you are not hundred percent sure. If you ask, you can avoid the mistake. So my advise is to all of you do not hesitate to ask if you are not sure about anything. These three things are significant to complete the new graduate nursing program successfully.

I wish all of you to have great success in your future endeavours. Thank you and good luck to you all.

REFERENCES

Blann, A 2014, 'Why do we test for urea and electrolytes?', *Nursing Times,* vol. 110, pp. 19- 21.

Burch, J 2013, 'Back to basics: how to care for different types of stoma', *Nursing and Residential Care,* vol. 15, no.10, pp.662- 665.

Caffsso, J 2015, *What are intramuscular injections?* Healthline.

Case-lo, C 2015, *what is subcutaneous injection?* Health Line.

Cayley, WE 2007, 'preventing deep vein thrombosis in hospital inpatients', *US National library of medicine national Institute of Health,* vol.335, no. 7611, pp. 147- 151.

CCU 2014, *'Commonly Used Cardiac Medications"* St Vincent's Hospital Sydney.

Craven, R & Hirnle, C 2003, *Fundamental of nursing: human health and function,* 4th edn, Lippincott Williams & Walkins.

Cretikos, M, Bellomo, R, Hillman, K, Chen, J, Finfer, S & Flabouris, A 2008, 'Respiratory rate: the neglected vital signs' *MJA,* vol.188, no.11.

DCRC 2014, Your Brain Matters, DCRC, Australia

http://yourbrainmatters.org.au/5-simple-steps/step-1-look-after-your-heart?gclid=CPG-tu20g80CFYeSvQodMqELvA.

DHHS 2014, *Transmission based precautions*, DHHS, Tasmania.

European Pressure Ulcer Advisory Panel and national Pressure Ulcer Advisory Panel (EPUAP/NPUAP) 2009, *Pressure Ulcer Prevention Quick Reference Guide*, EPUAP/NPUAP, Washington DC.

Farrell, M & Dempsey, J 2011, *Smeltzer & Bare's textbook of medical-surgical nursing*, 2nd edn, Wolters Kluwer/Lippincott Williams & Wilkins, Philadelphia.

Farrell, M 2005, 'Fluid and Electrolytes: Balance and Distribution', in M Farrell, S C. Smeltzer &B G. Bare (eds), *Smeltzer & Bare's Text Book of Medical Surgical Nursing*, Lippincott Williams & Wilkins, Brodway NSW, pp.253- 289.

Farrell, M 2005, 'Preoperative Nursing Management' in M Farrell (ed), *Smeltzer &Bare's Textbook of Medical Surgical Nursing*, Lippincott Williams & Wilkins, Broadway NSW, pp. 402-419.

Farrell, M 2005, 'Intraoperative Nursing Management' in M Farrell (ed), *Smeltzer &Bare's Textbook of Medical Surgical Nursing*, Lippincott Williams & Wilkins, Broadway NSW, pp. 421- 439.

Farrell, M 2005, 'Postoperative Nursing Management' in M Farrell (ed), *Smeltzer &Bare's Textbook of Medical Surgical Nursing*, Lippincott Williams & Wilkins, Broadway NSW, pp. 440 - 462.

L8 (SVPH) 2014, FB Chart for Nurses Module.

Levett-Jones, T, Hoffman, K, Dempsey, J, Jeong, S, Noble, D, Norton, C, Roche, J & Hickey, N 2009, 'The five rights of clinical reasoning: An educational model to enhance nursing students' ability to identify and manage clinically 'at risk' patients', *Nurse Education Today*, vol.3.

Kayilioglu, S, Dinc, T, Sozen, I, Bostanoglu, A, Cate, M & Coskun F 2015, 'Post-Operative Fluid Management', *World Journal of Critical Care Medicine*, vol. 4, no.3 pp. 192-201.

Maneval, R., Fowler, K., Kays, J., Mastrine, C., Boyd, T 2012 'The effect of high-fidelity patient simulation on critical thinking and clinical decision-making skills in new graduate nurses' *Journal of Continuing Nursing Education*, vol.43, no.3, pp. 125-134.

Maton, P & Burton, M 1999, 'Antacids revisited: a review of their clinical pharmacology and recommended therapeutic use', *Drugs*, vol. 57, no.6, pp. 855 -870.

Munckhof, W 2005, 'Antibiotics for surgical prophylaxis', *Australian Prescriber*, vol. 28, pp. 38 - 40.

Myers, BA 2004, *Wound management: principles and practice*, Prentice Hall: Upper Saddle River, New Jersey.

McGrath, J 2005, *You Inc, 1st, Australia*.

National Safety and Quality Health Service (NSQHS) 2012, *Standard 8 Pressure Injury*, NSQHS, Queensland, viewed 25 January 2015, < http://www.health.qld.gov.au/psu/safetyandquality/docs/pip-audit-def.pdf>.

National Institute for Health and Care Excellence (NIHCE) 2013, *Intravenous fluid therapy in adults in hospital*, NIHCE, UK, December2013, viewed1February2015, <http://www.nice.org.uk/guidance/cg174/chapter/introduction>.

New South Wales Health (NSWH) 2011, *Transition to Practice Emergency Nursing Program*, NSWH, North Sydney NSW.

NSWDH 2011, *Workplace culture framework*, NSWDH, North Sydney http://www.health.nsw.gov.au/workforce/Publications/workplace-culture-framework.pdf.

Northwest Regional Spinal Cord Injury System (NWRSCIS) 2009, *Skincare and pressure sores*, NWRSCIS, University of Washington, Washington DC, viewed 27th January 2015, http://sci.washington.edu/info/pamphlets/msktc-stages.asp.

Nursing and Midwifery Board of Australia (NMBA) 2006, *National competency standards for the registered nurse*, NMBA, January 2006, viewed 13th January 2015, < http://www.nursingmidwiferyboard.gov.au/Codes-Guidelines-Statements/Codes-Guidelines.aspx#competencystandards >.

Purser, K 2009, 'Wound dressing guidelines', *Royal United Hospital Bath NHS Trust*, vol.2, pp.6.

Saladin, K, S 2012, *Anatomy & Physiology: The unity of form and function*, 6th edn, 1221 Avenue of the Americas, N. Y.

Sanderson, M & Allison, EW 2007, 'Thyroidectomy: preoperative and postoperative nursing care', *The American journal of Nursing*, vol.39, no 3, pp. 244-248.

Shephard, A 2011, 'Measuring and Managing Fluid Balance', *Nursing Times*, vol.107, no.28, pp.12-16.

Staples, WD 1991, *Think like a Winner*, Pelican publishing company Inc., Louisiana.

Tiziani, A 2010, *Harvard's nursing guide to drugs*, 9th edn, Mosby, Sydney.

Peters, T & Robert H. Waterman, Jr 2004, *In Search of Excellence*, 1st, Profile Books, Great Britain.

Walker, J 2007, 'Patient preparation for safe removal of surgical drains art and science clinical skills', *Nursing standard*, vo. 21, no. 49, pp. 39-41.

Woodbury, 1 & De Ora, W 2008, *The Invisible Entrepreneur*, 1st, Quantum Dynamics, Australia.

World Health Organization (WHO) 2015, *WHO's pain relief ladder*, WHO, viewed 1 February 2015, < http://www.who.int/cancer/palliative/painladder/en/>.

World Health Organization (WHO) 2007, *Standard precaution in health care*, WHO, Switzerland.

Woodward, M 1999, 'Risk factors for pressure ulcers-can they withstand the pressures?', *Primary Intention*, vol. 52.

Printed in the United States
By Bookmasters